YOUR PET'S
SECRET
LANGUAGE

YOUR PET'S SECRET LANGUAGE

How to Understand It and Speak It

JHAN ROBBINS

Peter H. Wyden/Publisher

NEW YORK

YOUR PET'S SECRET LANGUAGE

Copyright © 1975 by Jhan Robbins

Library of Congress Cataloging in Publication Data

Robbins, Jhan.
    Your pet's secret language.

    Bibliography: p.
    1. Pets—Behavior. 2. Animal communication.
I. Title.
SF412.5.R6   001.5   75-703
ISBN 0-88326-085-9

243

Manufactured in The United States of America

Dedication

To Squibber, Eloise, Penrod, Nimrod, Agamemnon, Albert, Bachelor Bill, Pinky, Rusty, Willie, Shanty, Benny, Dee Dee, Dumas, Dungorten, Beaner, Ada, Fearless, Soaky, Brig, Cleo and all the other pets who have contributed so much love, understanding and happiness to their (sometimes uninformed) owners.

Acknowledgments

Dr. Michael Fox, Dr. Konrad Lorenz, Dr. Elisabeth Mann Borgese, Dr. Jacob Antelyes, Dr. John Lilly, Dr. Preston Holder, Dr. Joyce Wike, Dr. David Premack, Dr. Philip Haims, Dr. Sara Barnhart, Dr. Beatrice Gardner, Dr. Allen Gardner, Sallie Prugh, Cleveland Amory, Gillette Grilhé, Captain Arthur Haggerty, Lew Burke, Matthew Margolis, Barbara Austin, Herb Clement, Alice and Mike Haller, Manuel Mendez, Katherine Coke, Melida and John Marver, Flip and Sandy Saunders, Leon Wolfer, Angela and Ian Kennedy, Dorothy and Bob Weil, Gail Moreso, Joy McGinnis, Henry Spellman, Janie Greenberg, Lenore Faubel, Philip Chapman, Jr., Miriam Johnson, Martin Anderson, Selma Blassingame, Natalie Parnass, Dr. F. Dudley Klopfer, Dr. William Martin, Dr. Ronald Wilensky, Ada Maud Thompson, June Reno, Penny Robbins, Meg Simon, Teddy Wahl.

Contents

Introduction
by Cleveland Amory

The Fund for Animals, of which I am president, has as its proud slogan: "We speak for those who can't."

Now, it appears, animals not only can speak, they do speak. The trouble is we don't know how to listen.

This book tells us how. And don't think it is just the story of a few famous animals. They are here, yes: the story of the famous chimp "Washoe"; the story of "Buddy," Lew Burkes' German shepherd who not only goes on talk shows but talks on them; even the story of a primate who drove his trainer's automobile—at seventy miles an hour—and got a ticket.

But much more important, this is the story of *your* pet. Indeed, its's your ticket to getting more out of your relationship with your pet—both for you and for him.

Jhan Robbins has talked to dozens and dozens of pet owners who have actually talked to their pets—and vice versa. Before you know it, if you follow the instructions here, you will be able to do the same thing with your pet. Best of all, you will understand why the sheep-herder you read about here never scolds his dog in front of other dogs, or even in front of the sheep!

As for your cat, you will learn to know—and re-spect—its "four freedoms"; understand why it likes to watch a cowboy or a Western show on TV in prefer-ence to most animal shows. And you will finally have sympathy for the woman who says, "The myths about cats being untrainable are spread by dog owners."

Nor will you be limited here to dogs and cats. The author tells us that many scientists feel the greatest hope of "obtaining non-human communication da-ta"—they mean hearing an animal talk—lies in birds. And this means talk not just from parrots and canaries and mynah birds but from all kinds of birds—even lovebirds.

As for horses, well, a Harvard psychologist tells a story here to prove they're not bright. Some may not be—but neither are some Harvard psychologists. Believe it or not, you can communicate with your horse, but you will learn that you get best results if you use a Southern accent or a Western drawl. I can't wait till a state of Maine man reads that one.

Finally, Albert Payson Terhune says something here that, to me, says it all: "Too many owners confuse love with respect, or vice versa—they are not the same thing."

This book is about love—yes. But, just as important, it is about respect. And your pet needs both.

What I Believe

When I started the research for this book I believed that an intelligent and interested pet owner could learn to recognize when his animal was saying, **"I'm hungry,"** or **"I want out."** I also felt that the pet could learn commands for **"come," "sit," "stay,"** and master other simple signals. But I must admit that I was very skeptical when an owner claimed, "Prince understands nearly everything I say."

Now, many months later, and after observing hundreds of pets, talking to dozens of scientists, veterinarians, psychologists, trainers, zoo keepers, circus performers, perceptive pet owners, and others closely associated with animals, I have come to the conclusion that it's quite possible for the average man, woman or child to carry on effective two-way conversations with a pet, using both verbal and non-verbal language. I'm not claiming that you can debate the political motivation of Watergate with your dog or have your cat hold forth on the respective merits of Leonard Bernstein versus Pierre Boulez, but you certainly can discuss the pet's intended visit to the vet or tell the animal about your day at the office—and elicit meaningful responses.

My animal communication investigation took me to many sections of the country and soon revealed that dolphins and chimpanzees, whose ability to communicate has been so widely publicized, are not alone in understanding and using extensive vocabularies. Dr. Elisabeth Mann Borgese, an outstanding animal behaviorist (and daughter of Thomas Mann), told me, "The performances of dolphins and chimpanzees pale when compared to an ordinary household pet. . . ."

Fortunately, you don't have to be a scientist or undergo technical training to carry on these conversations. I witnessed meaningful communication between pets and people who had never completed grade school. It's not very hard. And here's how.

NOTE: I would like to apologize to the owners of female pets for the frequent use of "he." But it would have been very awkward indeed to have to say "he" or "she" every time I alluded to an animal.

J. R.

YOUR PET'S
SECRET
LANGUAGE

CHAPTER I

Science Discovers That Animals Can Talk

Humans are no longer unique. We must now concede that the last significant distinction that was ours and ours alone is rapidly vanishing—*language*. Until recently, students of human behavior pointed out that in this one important area man was superior to all other creatures because he possessed a highly developed system of verbal communication and that this unique ability set him apart. However, recent research shows that animal systems of communication contain most of the basic characteristics of human spoken language.

And why not? Animals do make distinctive sounds, and forms of silent communication have been recognized for a long time. Most of us know:

• Young and inexperienced mothers who quickly learn the meaning of their infants' cries and gestures.

• Deaf mutes who communicate solely by the use of hand signals.

• Ordinary men and women who habitually express themselves through nods, shrugs, winks, touches, and other motions.

• Travelers in strange lands who make themselves understood by resorting to pantomime.

Today, psychologists, veterinarians, trainers, and other professionals closely associated with animals are putting these facts to work and unveiling some startling feats of animal intelligence and linguistic ability.

In Paris, a dog and a cat have been trained to act as receptionists in the office of a busy animal practitioner. They greet incoming patients and escort them to seats. When the veterinarian needs an instrument, one of his "receptionists" is able to bring the correct one.

In Thailand, a monkey is employed as a bank teller, and when he detects a counterfeit coin he instantly reports his findings to the assistant manager.

Before you dismiss these incidents as outlandish, far-fetched, or as fairy tales, ask yourself: did you really ever expect to watch men walk on the moon? Dr. Henry Eyring, former president of the American Association for the Advancement of Science, said, "The universe is so complex that even the widest-ranging vision is at best partial and tentative. Each generation sets itself the task of reevaluation and reinterpretation, a quest for truth is unending."

Scientists are learning that today anything is possible—even the incredible (but true) story of the primate who drove his trainer's automobile at more than seventy miles an hour along a California road. The ape was halted by a state trooper and, as the astonished officer was writing out a ticket, the simian nonchalantly scratched his cheek, blinked his eyes, shook his head, and grunted. The trainer, who was sitting on the passenger side, knew what it all meant. The ape was pretending complete innocence and was saying, **"Who me? What did I do wrong?"** Despite the ape's driving skill, the trainer was eventually fined for allowing "other than a human being to operate a moving vehicle."

Animals' communicating ability isn't frequently tested in traffic, but other systematic, scientific methods are currently being used to teach them to "speak" and understand. Dr. Michael Fox, a veterinarian and associate professor of psychology at Washington University in St. Louis, told me, "It is quite possible for the owner of the average pet to carry on two-way conversations." Dr. Fox, who is recognized as one of the country's leading authorities on animal behavior, added, "The average pet owner doesn't realize the potential his animal has. There is an enriching experience and special joy in owning a communicating pet—both the animal and the owner will be happier because of it."

Americans love animals with a passion—and they actively show it. Currently, there are more than 100 million dogs and cats in the United States, plus an additional 20 million pet birds. It is estimated that 60 percent of American households have at least one animal in residence and that every year pet owners spend more than $2 billion just for feeding the pets commercially prepared food.

Agriculture Secretary Earl Butz commented on this fact and committed a politically explosive faux pas by suggesting whimsically that Americans could help feed the world's starving people by getting rid of 50 percent of all pets. Immediately, the secretary's statement drew a thunder of outraged cries. Typical was the comment of a dog owner in Milwaukee who said, "I plan to ship Butz half of my litter of poodles because I haven't the guts to destroy them. I suppose being a Washington bureaucrat gives you sufficient guts!" (Up to this writing the embittered lady hasn't followed through with her threat.)

In addition to the staggering food bill, Americans spend at least another $2 billion annually on veterinary care, grooming, pet accessories and services such as clothing, jewelry, cosmetics, health insurance, cemetery plots, professional pet sitters and walkers. . . .

If you live in Los Angeles and have $5,000 to spare it is now possible to buy your pet a diamond-studded collar, or if you can only splurge on $100 you can arrange to have your animal called for in a special limousine and driven to a pet restaurant that serves such delicacies as *Bisque Parisienne de meal wheat, Marcelle tenderloin steak bones* and *Ambrosia kibble crêpes suzette.*

There are simpler, less costly, and more effective and loving ways to make your animal happy. Scientists have discovered that communicating regularly with your pet produces gratifying and pleasurable effects on the pet and the owner, too.

In 1974 many of the nation's 30,000 veterinarians reported that their case loads had increased sharply and that worried pet owners sought their counsel more and more frequently. The same was true for obedience training schools: they, too, were flooded with concerned owners seeking assistance.

If you own a pet, such doctors and schools are often essential for its well-being, but can these professionals help you in learning how to converse with your animal? Can they furnish any techniques for communication short cuts? Can they implement any of the methods described in this book?

Yes, *but*—and the but is a powerful one—you must locate someone with adequate pet language knowledge and sufficient time to observe your animal for very extended periods indeed. And when you do, you have to be prepared to spend hundreds and hundreds of dollars to get the job done properly. Even if you are lucky and happen to locate such a professional—and have vast funds—the results won't be remotely as good as if you did the job yourself. Animal behaviorists have discovered that when it comes to teaching the ability to communicate, nobody—but nobody—can effectively and fully take the place of an attentive, well-loved owner. (The authorities have also found that household pets frequently refuse to make use of their skills in front of strangers.)

The art of communicating with animals is a new field. This is the first time that the state of knowledge in this field has been pulled together in one place and made usable for laymen. The fact that learning how to converse with your animal isn't very difficult may come as a surprise to many. So be it. At least it's a pleasant surprise. It does require time and patience but—blissfully—no money.

So don't look for applicable listings in the Yellow Pages of the telephone directory—there aren't any. And even if "experts" appeared under *P* for *Pet Language Training,* they would still perform the job with less than maximum results. This is one time when only you can accomplish the job at its best. Here are some pet owners who regularly converse with their animals.

• Fred Waterman, a carpenter in Raleigh, North Carolina, has reaped the special joy of carrying on two-way conversations with Beau, his part retriever, part poodle, part terrier. Mr. Waterman will tell Beau, "I'm expecting a letter from Michael—fetch the mail."

Immediately, there will be a shift in Beau's facial expression. His eyes will crinkle, he will appear to be smiling, and he will hold his head erect. Mr. Waterman knows that Beau is saying, **"I'll be glad to get the mail and I feel that today you'll get a letter from Mike."**

Beau will then run outdoors and intercept the postman. The mail carrier has covered the route for a long time and is aware that Mr. Waterman, a widower, looks forward eagerly to hearing from his son, Michael, a marine sergeant stationed in Spain. If indeed that day does produce a letter from Michael, the postman makes the happy announcement to the dog. Beau recognizes the delighted tone and promptly gathers the letter in his mouth, races indoors, lays the envelope at his owner's feet and gives not one but three joyous barks. Again Mr. Waterman knows what the dog is saying. Beau is telling him, **"It's come! It's come! It's come!"**

• Another happy twosome are Joan Cooper and her tiger-striped cat, Cleo. Ms. Cooper, who teaches third grade in a Texas private school, consistently communicates with her four-year-old feline. She often brings Cleo to class and tells her, "Find an empty desk."

The cat lifts up her head and Ms. Cooper notices that the eyes—which are slightly crossed—have widened and changed color. The cat miaows briefly; she is saying, **"Yes."**

As the cat locates a vacant seat the teacher adds, "And do be quiet!"

Hearing that command, Cleo stares solemnly, cocks her ears and once again miaows. But this time the miaowing is different—it is longer and mellower. Ms. Cooper understands. Mischievous Cleo, whose saucer eyes are now opened very wide, is saying, **"It'll be hard, but I'll try."**

• Ms. Rhoda Orloff of Seattle, Washington, also relishes the role of owning a communicating pet. For two years she has been carrying on conversations with Glenda, her cinnamon-colored Yorkshire canary. Every evening Ms. Orloff asks the bird, "What kind of day will tomorrow be?"

Glenda, who has gained the reputation for being an enthusiastic (if not infallible) weather prophet, immediately starts to sing. Ms. Orloff has learned to distinguish between the songs. One means, **"It will be cold"** and a higher-pitched version means, **"It will be hot."** If Glenda feels especially communicative she changes her tune, which translates to: **"It will be clear"** or, **"It will rain."** The bird's repertoire is vast and also includes, **"I am hungry," "I am thirsty,"** and **"I am lonely."**

The perceptive owner explains, "My Glenda's replies may not be in perfect King's English, but then she hasn't earned a Ph.D. at Oxford. However, her singing and body motions are clear enough for me."

Some readers may suspect by now that I toured the nation in search of super-dogs, super-cats and superbirds—the Einsteins of the animal world, in a manner of barking. *I did not.* Yes, some of the animals you will meet in these pages are brighter than their peers. No, there are no popular IQ tests for animals as yet, at least none that I value. But there is no question remaining in my mind that the acts of communication described here, taken in sum total, have well-documented, universal applicability. Which does not mean that somewhere there might not be some old dog who really can't be taught old tricks, let alone new ones. Yes, such a dog (or cat or bird) is possible, and I pray that he is not yours.

Most experiments revealing that human beings are not the only ones who possess the ability to speak are of recent vintage, and one of the pioneer projects was conducted in the 1940s by Dr. Karl von Frisch, a German biologist. He startled the scientific world by announcing that bees communicate with each other through a language that is all their own.

Dr. von Frisch discovered that by dancing, a bee communicates the direction and distance of food. The scientist put out bowls of sugar water, which bees regard as delicious dessert. As soon as the scout bee located the water it would fly back to its hive and tell the other bees of the discovery. This was done by a series of carefully scripted gyrations which Dr. von Frisch called "the waggling dance." The scout bee was saying, **"Food—come and get it! Fly in a southeasterly line and you will come to it!"**

If the food was nearby, one hundred yards or less, the bee would go through a fairly simple routine; if the food was farther away, the dance became more complicated. For example: a dance lasting two seconds meant that the food was a mile away. Dr. von Frisch was amazed at the bees' accuracy—their "language" was so exact that the scientists could go to the precise spot that the scout bee had indicated.

J. B. S. Haldane, one of the world's outstanding biologists, called the bee communication discovery "a landmark in human achievement comparable with Champollion's elucidating of hieroglyphics." Dr. von Frisch has since become a Nobel Laureate.

Another German scientist, Dr. Otto Koehler, of the University of Freiburg, contributed additional data along more sophisticated lines: *not only could animals give accurate directions, but they could also count.* He found that although animals may not have names for their numbers they can definitely count. Squirrels can count to seven; parakeets to six; pigeons to five.

Dr. Koehler's experiments were intricate, meticulously conducted, and were performed thousands of times before a report was issued. The scientist had discovered that animals translated a "heard" number into a "seen" one. A series of jars were placed side by side and each was marked with a different number of dots; then a drum was sounded. The results were startling. For example, if a squirrel (or parakeet or pigeon) heard four drum beats, the animal would select the jar with four dots; five drum beats, the jar with five dots. The animal would then lift off the top of the jar, knowing that a food reward was inside.

This capacity to learn a skill such as counting is not to be confused with the tricks taught to animals such as Roy Rogers' horse Trigger, who could "count" with his hoof. Such entertainment gimmicks can be drilled into animals by rote. Here I am talking about real intelligence and real comprehension.

Other animal communicating experiments followed: it was learned that rabbits thump their hind feet sharply on the ground to signify impending danger; a female duck transmits fear by jumping out of the water and uttering a very distinctive piercing cry; a finch is usually the first to spot trouble in the woods and passes the alarm on to other forest creatures by a series of honking sounds.

"All that you need to properly translate the animal's 'speech,'" says Dr. Henri Saypol, a French psychologist, "is patient observation." He adds, "And most people can afford this simple but important luxury if the desire is present."

The next series of research projects focused on primates because they bear the closest resemblance to man phylogenetically and it was thought therefore that they could be trained to master human speech. Scientists regard these experiments as some of the most significant in animal-man communication. In the 1950s Dr. Keith Hayes, a scientist at the Yerkes Regional Primate Research Center in Atlanta, Georgia, and his wife, Cathy, brought a tiny chimpanzee infant into their home. Viki, the chimp, was only three days old when she arrived and the Hayeses decided to raise her as an "only human child." They showered her with loads of love and care, yet, despite this lavish attention, the chimpanzee could learn only three human words by the time she was three years old. She hoarsely whispered, "**Mama**," "**Papa**," and "**Cup.**"

This venture was soon followed by what scientists refer to as "the chimp turning-point." Previous attempts to teach chimps to talk had met with slight success because simians lack the anatomy for speech. The larynx and other motor apparatus are there, but primates seem to possess little voluntary control over them. Therefore, Dr. David Premack, a professor of psychology at the University of California, decided to establish a non-vocal line of communication. He selected Sarah, a five-year-old chimpanzee, as his subject. Dr. Premack and his associates decided to use small pieces of plastic that varied in shape and color. Each piece stood for one word within the following categories: objects, names, colors, food, adjectives, and adverbs. A strip of magnetized metal on the back of the plastic allowed the piece to be easily attached to a slate that was referred to as a "language board."

At first, Dr. Premack or his associates would put a banana on the table and watch as Sarah snatched the fruit and ate it. This routine continued until one day, a piece of plastic—a word—was introduced. This time, Sarah had to place the piece on the language board before she got the banana. Sarah soon learned that this was a game and began to enjoy it. The scientist then decided to introduce new words, and again the results were impressive.

Sarah was then given two words but only one piece of fruit, to see whether she could match the correct word with the food. She was generally successful in this test. After some weeks Dr. Premack began lessons in sentence structure. Again, Sarah proved to be an apt student and actually formed sentences. **"Apple red"** meant "The apple is red." Some sentences were more complicated: **"Mary give fig Sarah."**

Eventually, Sarah learned more than 130 words. Among them were these verbs: *prefer, close, insert, smoke, peel.* And these colors: *yellow, green, orange, red, blue.* And these foods: *banana, fig, cracker, peanut butter, jam.* And these objects: *table, shoe, paint brush, flashlight, broom.*

Sarah lived under standard laboratory conditions: wire cage and cement block walls. Her exposure to humans and to her special training was largely limited to the one hour of language practice which she received five days a week. However, Dr. Premack intends to erect a new compound for Sarah and her chimpanzee friends. The chimps will then be given more freedom and will have the opportunity to wander into a special learning center where language lessons and rewards will be available whenever they are interested.

To cynics who doubt that Sarah understands language, Dr. Premack says, "She understands well enough to teach her teachers. During a preposition test one day, Sarah, who became restless, gave one of my associates what amounted to a sentence completion test. Sarah put up a partial statement on one side of the language board [A is on . . .] and then arranged alternate answers on the other side. Sarah would point to each possible answer, and my associate's task—and it took her a while to figure out what Sarah wanted—was to nod when Sarah pointed to the right one.

" 'The little devil would pass by the solution quickly and try to trick me into making a mistake,' my associate reported."

Dr. Premack eventually hopes to adapt the same communication method that he used with Sarah and apply it to humans who have trouble learning language. In the meantime, he has found out a great deal about an animal's linguistic abilities—and he believes they are nothing short of staggering.

While Dr. Premack was experimenting with Sarah and her language board, two other pioneering scientists were attempting to establish non-vocal communication with a chimpanzee by using the language of the deaf, American Sign Language (ASL). This system of communication was developed for humans who can't hear the spoken word and consists of a set of hand gestures, each corresponding to an individual word. For example:

Cat. The thumb and index finger come together near the corner of the mouth and are moved outward, representing the cat's whiskers.

Think. Fingers on the right hand are extended and then placed against the forehead.

Smell. The palm is held in front of the nose and moved slightly upward several times.

Doctors Beatrice and Allen Gardner, a husband-and-wife team of psychologists at the University of

Nevada, decided to use the ASL system on Washoe, an eight-month-old female chimpanzee. The Gardners raised Washoe almost as if she were their own child. Washoe was quartered in a lavish, fully-equipped 24-foot-long house trailer (unlike Sarah's austere laboratory) located behind the Gardner home. The two psychologists or their resident assistants spent most of the day and night with the young chimp. They adhered to a simple rule: *"Use no language except ASL in Washoe's presence."* Sounds were permitted, but no spoken words.

Washoe was one year old in June 1966 when actual language instruction began; at that age her development and her needs were much like those of a human baby. She slept a great deal and had just begun to crawl. But soon after her first year Washoe started to associate gestures with activities. Her teachers taught her the sign for *more* in the context of tickling, romping, and wrestling. Washoe loved to rough-house.

Then they taught her the sign for *open,* using doors in the house trailer. She soon extended its use to apply to all doors, drawers, the refrigerator and, finally, to water faucets.

Early in 1967 Washoe began to form phrases. If she was thirsty, she made the symbol for **"give me"** and then added the one for **"drink."** Soon she was able to differentiate between similar objects. If all she wanted was a drink of water she gave only the gesture for **"drink":** thumb in the mouth, fingers drawn into a fist. But if she craved soda pop, she prefaced the **"drink"** signal with that for **"sweet":** a quick touching of the tongue with her fingertips. She was judged to have learned a sign if she used it of her own accord, and in a proper fashion, for fifteen days.

In April 1967, less than a year after her training began, she produced her first combination of signs, a kind of sentence. As Washoe learned nine or ten signs she started stringing them together in sets of two or three, much as small children learn to combine words. She was taught some of these combinations by her trainers, but others she made up herself.

A favorite was, **"Give me tickle."**

Increasingly, Washoe seemed to understand the gestures of others and she extended her ability to express them herself. One day in 1969, Dr. Roger Fouts, then a graduate student who worked with Washoe, told her in sign language that there was a large dog outside and it would harm her—all in symbols whose meaning she had been taught. He was telling Washoe a deliberate lie, but it disturbed her as much as the threat of a bogeyman might frighten a child. Her hair stood up and she was greatly upset. Since no physical clue was present—such as the scent of a real dog outside or fearful expressions on Dr. Fouts' part—psychologists concluded from Washoe's actions that she believed the information that her human handler was telling her. And when she was asked whether she wanted to go outside and play, an activity that she normally would have enjoyed, Washoe vigorously gave the gesture for **"no."**

Washoe went to the University of Oklahoma along with Dr. Fouts, after the latter had gained his doctorate at the University of Nevada. There is a small colony of chimpanzees at Oklahoma's Institute for Primate

Studies undergoing similar ASL training, and it was thought that Washoe would benefit from a transfer to the Norman campus with its better-equipped facilities. Washoe approved the move and her vocabulary grew to more than 175 words.

Today, in the Oklahoma experiment, under the direction of Dr. William B. Lemmon, a group of chimps are communicating with their teachers through hand signals. Lucy, a seven-year-old chimpanzee, is one of the brighter students. She was raised from birth in the home of psychology professor Maurice Temerlin. Lucy knows signs for household objects, clothing, toys, personal names, verbs and adjectives. She can execute many different requests consisting of two or three words—such as **"hug Lucy,"** or **"catch ball."**

There is recent evidence that Lucy can invent signs of her own to describe objects she would dearly like to have. Scientists at the Oklahoma research center observed her bending her index finger into a hook shape and touching it to her neck. Lucy had never been taught a sign similar to that, but the startled psychologists soon realized that it referred to her leash —and that Lucy was asking to be taken out for a walk.

The youngest student in the University of Oklahoma's remarkable project is Salome. At four months of age, she already uses two symbols: **"drink"** (thumb touching mouth) and **"food"** (four fingers touching mouth).

Classes start each day at 8:30 A.M. After a quick hug and a romp, the chimp and teacher settle down to work. The lessons are kept as informal and varied as possible. The chimps usually become quickly bored with the drill and would much rather be chased around the room, so they constantly interrupt the silent exchange of signals with insistent demands for a tickle. Every ten or twenty minutes the teacher and chimp break off for a relaxing tussle.

At the Yerkes Regional Primate Research Center in Atlanta, Georgia, scientists are delighted with the progress of Lana, a four-year-old chimpanzee, who has learned enough of a modified English to converse with people through a computerized keyboard. Although the computers and other equipment necessary for Lana's progress are complicated, their operation is simple. In Lana's room there is a machine with seventy-five buttons, each bearing a distinctive symbol: a triangle, a line, or a circle. Each button stands for one word.

When Lana presses a button, a typewriter outside her room prints the equivalent word in English. If Lana presses the buttons for **"Please, machine, give me a piece of apple,"** a vending machine serves up a piece of apple. Lana can also ask for water, milk, the opening of a window, or the playing of music.

Some of Lana's conversations are quite sophisticated. Here's part of a recent one she had with Timothy V. Gill, a doctoral student who is the chimpanzee's friend and teacher:

GILL: *What color of this?*
LANA: **Color of this orange.**
GILL: *Yes.*
LANA: **Tim, give cup which is red.**
GILL: *Yes.* (Gave her a red cup which she tossed away.)
LANA: **Tim, give apple which is green.** (Lana frequently confused orange and green.)

GILL: *No apple which is green.*
LANA: **Tim, give apple which is orange.**

Not only can Lana ask for concrete objects by the names she has been taught, but she can also ask for objects whose names she doesn't know. Lana is not a passive learner and has begun asking to be taught things she wants to know. Often, she will inquire: **"What's this?,"** and **"What's that?"**

Now the scientists are waiting for some of these chimpanzees to produce children of their own. When they do, it is hoped that the chimps will start teaching their offspring how to communicate with humans.

Can non-humans pass on their language ability from generation to generation? Experts working closely with bottlenose dolphins—warm-blooded and air-breathing mammals—believe that not only is this possible, in the case of dolphins it is very probable. The dolphin, whose intelligence may well rival that of humans, has probably been communicating for thousands of years. Aristotle wrote in the fourth century B.C., "This creature [the dolphin] has a voice."

Recently, actor George C. Scott starred in a popular movie called *The Day of the Dolphin,* whose dramatic action was based on two-way conversations between dolphins and human beings. The film was based on a research project being conducted by Dr. John C. Lilly, director and founder of the Communication Research Institute located in the Virgin Islands. Dr. Lilly is a doctor of medicine whose initial interest in dolphins was triggered by the mammal's huge and complex brain.

The brain of the dolphin is 40 percent larger than man's, and the cortex, the layer of gray matter, is just as complex. The normally developed human brain contains some 13 billion interconnecting neurons and 65 billion glia cells to actuate the speaking and writing functions. A dolphin brain contains an even larger number of these crucial elements.

When Dr. Lilly started working with live dolphins he became impressed with their extreme intelligence and started thinking seriously about the possibility of inter-species communication. Eventually he learned that dolphins definitely possess a vocabulary:

• Jaws snapping shut means: **"Stop what you are doing."**

• A crisp bark: **"I'm afraid."**

• A double whistle: **"Help, I'm in serious trouble."**

• A yelping sound: **"I'm looking for a mate."**

In one of Dr. Lilly's initial experiments he placed a microphone over a dolphin's blowhole in order to amplify the sounds that the dolphin was emitting. Dr. Lilly felt that the dolphin was making sounds that resembled laughter. But when tape recordings of the sounds were played and studied, Dr. Lilly and his associates made an unexpected detection. "We discovered," he says, "that the dolphin had been mimicking some of the things I'd been saying."

Perhaps the most amazing experience Dr. Lilly has had with dolphins' ability to mimic human speech came as long ago as 1960, when one of the dolphins, named Lizzie, became seriously ill. One evening when the scientist insisted on personally tending Lizzie, he was urged by an associate to come in for dinner.

"**It's six o'clock!**" he was suddenly told. Someone other than his associate had made the statement, but there was no one else there—*except the dolphin!*

"Lizzie," says Dr. Lilly, "came out very loudly with a 'humanoid' sentence, the meaning of which, if any, has puzzled several of us since. It may have been a poor copy of 'It's six o'clock!' But I was caught first by another 'meaning.' It sounded to me like, 'This is a trick!' with a peculiar hissing accent. Other people have since heard the tape and have come to the same conclusion." Lizzie was known to possess a great sense of humor, and she may have been actually trying to trick Dr. Lilly.

The work of communicating with dolphins moves ahead—and very often it produces startling results. Recently in Florida a group of the animals were taught to harmonize and have been organized into a barbershop quartet. They may not perform at Lincoln Center, but their quacks, barks, and whistles are usually in tune. In another Florida aquarium, Sam, a precocious five-year-old dolphin, made clicking noises that sounded like, "**I ache! Rub my back!**" Sam's comment didn't seem incredulous to his keeper, who knew his charge was both a hypochondriac and garrulous.

Even serious scholars no longer dismiss such incidents because by now there are reams of scientific data attesting to conversations between non-humans and man.

Rabbits are the heroes in the bestseller *Watership Down.* The animals' behavior is consistent with the laws of nature, yet each rabbit is portrayed as a distinctive individual. The book is enjoying a phenomenal success and many readers have said that the animals' "human" behavior ceases to appear amazing after the first few pages and the fact that rabbits carry on conversations isn't shocking.

"Why should it be?" asked one British reviewer. "After all, animals observe man consistently—the time has arrived for us to do the same."

A great deal of the scientific material in *Watership Down* was drawn from a remarkable book by Ronald M. Lockley, entitled *The Private Life of the Rabbit.* Its author, a distinguished lapine biologist, believes that rabbits communicate in human ways quite frequently. "The scream-squeal of a rabbit in distress," he says, "is like that of a [human] child in extreme pain. . . . there are many similarities."

Even plants are engaged in communication. Another bestselling book, *The Secret Life of Plants,* assures gardeners that plants thrive when they hear the human voice. Not only does the owner's conversation make them flourish, but often the plants reply. Botanists are puzzled by this amazing discovery that seems to transcend all the physical laws hitherto recognized. However, the scientists are flexible enough to accept the authenticity of these "strange" events in communication that are reported with increasing frequency.

In Tokyo, Dr. Ken Hashimoto, chief of research for the Fuji Electronic Industries, has taught his cactus to solve simple mathematical problems. Dr. Hashimoto, who is also an expert in lie detection for the Japanese police, will ask a plant: "How much are two and two?" Soon after the query, the cactus makes a definite sound which Dr. Hashimoto records. Then he transposes the cassette into a graph. The answer then becomes clearly visible: *four distinct peaks!*

A legal typist in Toledo, Ohio, who is partially deaf, has trained her viburnum to inform her whenever the telephone rings. When the plant hears the phone ringing it droops slightly and returns to the original position when the owner answers it.

A prize-winning *Pravda* reporter visited the Timirayzev Academy in Moscow and wrote, "Before my very eyes a barley sprout literally cried out when its roots were plunged into hot water."

Dr. Elisabeth Mann Borgese, consultant at the University of California's Center for the Study of Democratic Institutions and also to the Encyclopedia Britannica, isn't surprised by any of these bizarre-sounding incidents. Dr. Borgese, who has conducted many serious experiments in animal communication, has herself accumulated massive evidence documenting the fact that the language barrier between man and beast has been broken.

"The scientific evidence which is piling up," she says, "should convince even the most pragmatic person that animals can talk. Experiments with bees, chimpanzees, dolphins, and others have proven that they do frequently. *However, their performances pale when compared to ordinary pets, who are usually thinking animals."* Dr. Borgese adds, *"I am certain that humans can converse with their pets. . . . I do regularly!"*

The drive toward pet-animal understanding is fed by psychological needs of long standing. We seem to have a great desire to endow our pets with human qualities. From childhood on animals play an important part in our lives, and we want our children and grandchildren to experience similar delights. Joyfully, we recommend books to them that display a veritable zoo of animals who dispense wisdom, manage entire households, raise children, and communicate with humans all over the place. The children love Ernest Seton Thompson's "yaller" dog, Wully, Albert Payson Terhune's faithful canine, Lad, or Beatrix Potter's Peter Rabbit. We regale them with Hugh Lofting's happy adventures of Dr. Dolittle and his piglet, Gab-Gab; his dog, Jip; and his housewifely duck, Dab-Dab. We can never forget "Puss 'n Boots" or "The Owl and the Pussycat." We're pleased when our youngsters want to see a Mickey Mouse film instead of a Frankenstein monster movie.

A. A. Milne, the British author of *Winnie the Pooh*, may have best explained why we like to think of animals as miniature humans when he said, "I had always been led to believe that most animals conduct themselves in exemplary fashion, and rarely do anything evil. When my son, Christopher Robin, wanted to listen to bedtime stories I naturally invented tales about harmless talking pets. I suppose I was trying to shield him from real people in the real world as long as possible."

CHAPTER II

Necessary Tools for Pet Communication

"Language, like the 'good' child, is often seen but not heard," says Dr. Jacob Antelyes, a Queens County, New York, veterinarian and popular columnist for *Modern Veterinary Practice.* "Unfortunately, we lose a great deal of what is being said simply by not being attentive. A good part of our conversation is frequently non-vocal and, unless we are observant, much of the language just vanishes into thin air."

The relatively new science of *kinesics* deals with this non-vocal communication and is based on the behavioral patterns of speaking without words, the signals popularly known as body language: the agitated movement of the fingers, the twitch at the corner of the mouth, the furtive shifting of the eyes, often reveal the individual's true feelings. You can usually detect the phony smile of the man who says, "I don't like her at all," while at the same time shaking his head up and down.

For further proof that silent language is in constant

use, just observe working men and women around you who find it essential to communicate non-verbally: the traffic officer directing automobiles at a busy intersection; the airplane mechanic who guides planes to and from the runway; the boss of a derrick crew who tells his operators when to lower and raise their cranes; the music conductor who leads the orchestra through subtle shadings of tempo and sound levels just by waving a baton; the baseball umpire who "calls" balls and strikes. All these people normally operate in sophisticated ways—yet in almost total silence—and their message are often clearer than speech.

Marcel Marceau and other professional pantomimists have spent a lifetime refining their art by bypassing verbal language and conveying messages to audiences without regard to age or national culture. Scientists have found that animals do exactly the same thing —only they often do it better, since mimicry is their chief language. *Kinesics* is vastly more important to your pets than it is to you, because the animals have to rely almost completely on body movements and facial expressions for comprehension, especially when they communicate with each other.

Unlike humans, animals don't lie, and they clearly telegraph their thoughts as they move their faces, open their mouths, swish their tails. Every motion, despite its subtlety, reveals information in a continuous flow—and the animals have a great deal of excellent equipment with which to transmit their thoughts.

For example, the lips and cheeks of the dog are moved by nine different muscles; the ear by sixteen. The expressions of his eyes are also used for transmitting information: partially closed eye often means puzzlement and the widening of the pupil is frequently a sign of irritation.

The eyes of the cat are the largest and most expressive of any animal in relation to its body weight. The field of vision of the cat is exceptional—it extends to 280 degrees while a binocular field is only 130 degrees. The cat's ears contain nearly thirty muscles, more than four times as many as in the human ear. The whiskers enable the cat to judge distance. If they bend back they're saying, "**I won't move!**"

The ears of the bird are not as obvious as those of the cat or dog, but a close observer will notice that many birds flick them constantly. Usually, a rapid flicking indicates a desire for food, and, when the ear movement slows down, it may be a sign of contentment. The eyes of the average bird are extremely sensitive and accurate. Just how accurate the bird's eyes are was reported by Professor Richard Herrnstein of Harvard University. He trained pigeons to look at 35-mm color slides and to peck at all human beings present in the picture. Sometimes the people in the slides were visible far in the distance, sometimes they were almost covered up.

"The precision of the animals was amazing," says Dr. Herrnstein. "More than once we found that we had misclassified a picture, either failing to see a hidden person or seeing one where there was none, only to be corrected by our pigeons."

How can we take advantage of the animal's obvious desire to communicate with man? Are there particular steps we can take to enable us to carry on conversations with our pets? *There certainly are!*

Again and again I found that three tools are essential for effective two-way conversations. If you want to converse successfully with your pet, I was told, you should be prepared to offer:

1. A *reward* for good performance.

2. An ability to make the pet realize that *affection* is always present in your heart and mind.

3. Large amounts of *patience.*

These three components of animal communication are often referred to as RAP. Most of the scientists who conducted the experiments discussed in the previous chapter used large measures of RAP. Sarah, the talkative chimpanzee who was raised by Dr. Premack, responded best when she was rewarded with something she liked—a banana or an orange. Washoe was fully aware that the Gardners were extremely fond of her. Dr. Lilly learned that when working with dolphins it was necessary to be very patient—his experiments were repeated over and over.

Psychiatrists and psychologists who treat humans often use behavior modification to help their patients. Part of the theory behind this treatment is that if a person does something positive and is promptly rewarded, he will do it again. Behavior modification has proved to be very effective with animals, too.

Sometimes the *reward* seems outlandish, as it does in this heart-warming story told to me by a barber in Philadelphia. He kept a canary in his small shop to entertain his customers while he cut their hair. Although the barber had a cage for the bird he often let her fly around loose. Occasionally, she perched on a customer's cheek or head, interrupting a shave or haircut.

"She knew what she was doing," said the barber, "but she'd stare at you, wiggle her beak, and break out in a joyous song. I'd studied her long enough to know that it was her way of saying *à la* Ben Bernie: **'Is everybody happy?'**

"However, when I first bought Galli—I named the canary Galli-Curci in honor of that great opera soprano—my Galli-Curci refused to sing! I tried everything to encourage her. I bought some records of other canaries singing (it was supposed to give her ideas) but no dice. I was told that another live bird would definitely teach her how to sing, so I rented a canary from a pet shop and the proprietor guaranteed 100 percent that my bird would sing, but again she refused. I know a lot of songs from operas and I sang to her, but that, too, didn't have any effect. She'd puff her neck out and shake her beak. I knew it meant, 'No!' That beak was almost as big as mine—one of my customers, a college professor, called it *'a cathedral type of beak.'*

"I offered Galli all kinds of bird goodies as rewards for singing: egg biscuit, celery, dandelion. She didn't want any of them. I was prepared to be stuck with a non-singing canary, but then one day an organ grinder came into my shop with his trained monkey. When the man started to play his instrument and the little monkey stretched out his hand for some coins, Galli suddenly flew toward the monkey and landed on his head. She balanced there a few seconds, then bent down and pecked him with her beak—it was definitely a kiss. Then she burst into a song! As long as I live, I'll remember that day; I was so overjoyed that I gave the organ grinder a free haircut!

"I was smart enough to realize that the little monkey's presence was the *reward* that made Galli sing. I encouraged the organ grinder to visit my shop every day. It was near his territory, so he and the monkey did visit. I told this to Galli and she'd primp while waiting for their arrival; she'd smooth out her feathers and look real nice. She sure had a crush on that monkey, but one day the organ grinder came in alone and announced sadly that the monkey had died. Instantly, Galli seemed to know what he was saying. The organ grinder soon got a new monkey, but it wasn't the same—Galli refused to sing. Three months later, she, too, died, I'm sure from a broken heart."

Affection, the second tool, means letting an animal know that you are glad the pet is part of the household. That doesn't mean that he should be made a *leading* member of the family, but it is vital simply to let him know that you like him.

You may think, "He's only an animal and can't possibly be aware of how I feel." But he does! And if he suspects that you hold him in a poor light, you can forget about conducting two-way conversations—he just will refuse to cooperate and might not even pay attention to your one-way communications.

A saleswoman I talked to in Newark, New Jersey, who had just learned that her services were no longer wanted because of the business recession, told me: "I'm going home to cry on my cat's shoulder. Well, maybe not her shoulder, it's rather narrow, but I'm sure she'll be very sympathetic when she hears I've been fired.

"It wasn't always that way. I'd always thought that cats were good for one thing only and that was to catch mice. I live in an old house and there are plenty of rodents to make a real tasty meal. The farther away the cat stayed from me, the better I liked it. If anyone had told me that I could talk to my cat I'd have called for the booby wagon real quick, but my cat seemed to have other ideas. She'd look at me with a curious kind of sad face that almost said, **'Why do you always ignore me? Don't you think I'm nice?'**

"So what could I do? I began to pet her—maybe just once or twice a day. Darned if she didn't go for that. They say that cats are loners, well, that cat sure loved the petting, so I did more of it and then still more. Pretty soon, her expression changed to sheer delight. The next thing I knew she'd jump up into my lap and lick my hands. I'd heard that cats like to be scratched behind their ears, so I did that. My cat is different, though. She didn't go for that at all—she prefers to have her back scratched.

"I suppose that deep down I'm a real softie. I started saying kind things to her like, 'What a nice pussycat you are!,' or 'That was real elegant the way you ate your dinner all up!' *How* you say it, I found out, is very important. I've been told that for a woman I have an unusually low voice and I've had to learn to raise it when I'm speaking to the cat. She knows when I'm bawling her out or praising her, just by the tone of my voice. Today we've become great friends. Like I told you, when she hears I was fired she'll comfort me and then she'll want to scratch the boss' eyes out!"

Herb Clement, former director of the Staten Island Zoo in New York, confirms this attitude: "The tone of voice is very significant. I've discovered that one can address an animal in dulcet tones while using derogatory words, but the animal will take its cue from the sound and purr contentedly. Often a dog who is trained to *sit* when the word is uttered in a commanding tone will not do so when the same word is murmured softly as a question. The dog may be puzzled by it and look at the owner as if expecting a clarifying command because he cannot understand the tone."

The last RAP implement is *patience,* and I was told very frequently that the successful pet owner needs an almost limitless reservoir of it. Jack Levinson, a prize-winning insurance agent in Dayton, Ohio, certainly qualifies on this count but he told me that it didn't come easy.

"I'm required to have plenty of patience," he said, "with my customers, my wife, my mother, my kids, even my landlord. Who has any left for a dog? The answer is . . . M–E! But I learned it in a most difficult way."

Levinson is a distinguished and sensitive-looking man. I can see why his customers have confidence in him and why he was given an award for selling a great many policies. He is lean, just over six feet tall, and his gray hair is frosty white at the temples. Pince-nez eyeglasses dangle across his vest.

"We have a German shephard whose name is Nannie," he told me. "Nannie offers some measure of protection and you certainly need lots of that around here. She's four years old but at times appears to look more like four months—she was the runt of the litter and the poor thing never really grew properly. We feed her a great deal, but it hasn't helped her stature.

"What she lacks in size, however, she more than makes up in sheer guts. Let anyone lay a hand on me and she immediately begins to growl. She never bites except on command. Two and a half years ago it was somewhat different—that's when she bit my neighbor as he was reaching for his garden hose to water the lawn. Nannie thought that he was picking up something to strike me with and lunged for him.

"I tried to stop her, but it was too late. Her teeth were already clamped on the poor man's hand. We had to quarantine her, even though she had had a rabies shot—there was a royal fuss and something just had to be done.

"Stopping Nannie from biting innocent people wasn't easy. It required perseverance and determination from both of us. Before his death, my father had been a tailor and my mother still had one of his stuffed mannequins. I took it and used it on Nannie. I'd pretend it was a real person and that I was about to be attacked; the first fifty times Nannie went for the stuffed dummy, but on the fifty-first occasion, she just growled and backed off. Patience had paid off. Currently, she won't do anything until I give the word, 'Attack!'

"It was the same way with words I wanted her to recognize. I'd show her a copy of *Atlantic* or *Harper's* and say, 'Magazine.' I'd repeat it incessantly and now when I tell her to 'fetch the magazine' she knows exactly what I want her to do. But it took patience, lots of it.

"The fascinating part about my using *patience* to teach Nannie is that it's rubbed off on my dealings with others. Not that I joined the million-dollar-insurance-policy club overnight, but the truth is I really think I have more forbearance than ever before—so now both my dog and I are more tranquil!"

While animal behaviorists insist that almost anyone can learn to carry on two-way conversations with a pet, you don't have to take the experts' word for it. In the following chapters, pet owners themselves will tell you just how they did it.

CHAPTER III

How Dogs Communicate

"Dogs, next to humans, are probably the most domesticated creatures on the face of the earth," says Captain Arthur Haggerty, former commanding officer of the army's K-9 Corps and currently director of the world's largest school for dog trainers. Captain Haggerty feels that dogs have voluntarily entered into a partnership with man—and that man has benefited tremendously from the close association. He points out: "Dogs don't lie, don't deceive, and never, never camouflage their emotions. Once you've learned to interpret the dog's expressions and movements you'll be able to understand his intentions forever!"

This man-dog partnership has existed for thousands of years, and many of the authorities with whom I talked believe that the relationship started when early tribesmen singled out the Asiatic wolf, one of the smallest members of the wolf family, and began to tame him. Others told me that the jackal or the coyote was the "original" dog; and still other serious students of canine behavior stoutly maintained that the dog has always been a species unto himself. Despite the controversy regarding the dog's true ancestry, authorities agree that the domesticated dog we know today is an ideal animal—loyal, loving, playful—and could hardly avoid being adopted by humans all over the world.

Migration played an important role in the development of canine life. It has long been considered highly fashionable to possess a dog of foreign origin. When the monarchy was still prevalent in the world, ranking kings or queens rarely allowed themselves to be painted or photographed without a "foreign" dog at their sides:

• King Louis XIV of France owned several Great Pyrenees that were bred by Spanish shepherds.

• Queen Victoria of England had a Borzoi that was a cross between an Arabian greyhound and a collie.

• Emperor Haile Selassie of Ethiopia owned a pair of Papillons.

In the United States "foreign" dogs have often graced the White House:

• Calvin Coolidge owned a white collie from northern Scotland.

• Franklin D. Roosevelt had a Scotch terrier

• John F. Kennedy had a Welsh terrier.

• Richard M. Nixon owned a Spanish cocker spaniel. (Some people believe that Checkers, the cocker spaniel, helped prolong Nixon's political career.) At Checkers' death Nixon brought three foreign dogs to the White House: a French poodle, a Yorkshire terrier, and an Irish setter.

Dr. Grover Allen, a zoologist and anthrolopogist at Harvard University, says that in our own country dogs owned by the early Indians probably arrived from Asia along with roving human beings. The American Indian treated the animal with a mixture of awe and savagery. Dr. Joyce Wike, a sociology professor at Nebraska Wesleyan University, made a detailed study of American Indians and their pets. She found that the elders in many tribes firmly believed the dogs to be reincarnations of the deceased. The Indians treated them accordingly—dogs that were believed to have been despicable enemies in a former life were kicked and abused; dogs who were thought to be honorable ancestors were deeply revered and received constant homage.

Dr. Wike told me about her visit to one reservation where she saw a small, brown and white mongrel enjoying great luxury. When she inquired why the dog was being treated so royally, she received an instant reply to her naive question: "Why, to do less would be very disrespectful—in a former life the dog was Chief Shooting Star!"

The early tribesmen spent months and sometimes years developing dogs into useful tribal helpers. They discovered that the animal made an excellent hunter and watchman. Because of superior hearing and sense of smell, a dog became aware of the presence of a strange person or animal long before his human owner did. The resulting barking and canine facial expressions may have been the first step in dog-to-man communication.

The second step probably came when humans learned that dogs also make ideal herders because just a small number of simple commands actually enable a dog to take excellent care of sheep or cattle. This step was followed by breeding dogs for special qualities.

Today, the leading categories and their talents as communicators are:

Working Dogs

Boxer. Has a very expressive face and the owner can easily detect changes. However, because of inbreeding the boxer is often high-strung and requires great patience.

Collie. Very even and easy disposition and seldom needs more than a few weeks to make known his likes and few dislikes. Collies love infants and seem to understand the meaning of many incoherent (to humans) baby sounds.

Doberman pinscher. He is very eager to please the owner and will often deliberately repeat movements to make certain his master knows what he is saying. His motto appears to be: "Look and listen!"

German shepherd. Trainers claim that dogs of this breed make the most apt pupils because of their super-intelligence. Although shepherds supposedly turn on their masters, this is usually the result of faulty communication. If you are using the shepherd as a guard it is essential that you give clear and concise commands to get your wishes carried out. Instant praise or rewards should follow.

St. Bernard. Children seem to understand them quicker than adults, so when in doubt you might check with your five-year-old daughter. St. Bernards seem to slobber constantly. Sometimes the foaming conveys a specific message and only careful observation will reveal its significance.

Sporting Dogs

Golden retriever. A very friendly breed that is usually very anxious to please the owner, but unless these dogs are watched carefully their movements are often mis-interpreted. When you finally understand them they will respond immediately—which is why they are used as seeing-eye dogs.

Labrador retriever. They communicate efficiently and eagerly by swishing their tails and by up and down movements of the ears. They're telling you something —and it's usually easy to find out what that is.

Irish setter. They are often extremely stubborn dogs and therefore great patience on the part of the owner is required. Any word or phrase should be repeated over and over.

Cocker spaniel. It's best to begin communication lessons with these dogs at an early age, yet they disprove the old cliché that you can't teach old dogs new tricks; owners have reported success even at the age of fifteen.

English setter. This is probably the easiest-going of all breeds and it therefore requires the owner's extra special effort to encourage them to communicate. It's not that they lack the capability; often they are just too lethargic. So be prepared to work a little harder.

Hounds

Bassett. They exhibit very expressive faces, but close observation is required to notice subtle changes. Owners should pay strict attention to their long, floppy ears, which often reveal a distinct message.

Basenji. This barkless dog is almost completely non-verbal, but makes up for being quiet by possessing an almost human face that gives off many human-like expressions. Basenji owners should pay special heed to enunciating each word distinctly.

Dachshund. Extensive patience is required, but the results are gratifying—almost total communication. This dog craves affection and the owner should be prepared to extend lavish praise for even the slightest "proper" performance.

Beagle. Use a minimum of force, since this dog is very stubborn and will resent interference. This is one time when owner patience is ultra-necessary. Offer praise when the dog cooperates, but *do not* ever reward a bad job.

Afghan. They seem to be aware of their regal appearance and expect the owner to constantly speak of it. They seem to cooperate more when you do so. This is one breed that can be taught new words in late adulthood. Try never to leave the Afghan completely unattended—he craves company.

Terriers

Fox terrier. This breed is capable of emitting a wide variety of sounds and communicates this way constantly. Barks, whines, and yelps usually have special meanings—observe carefully.

Airedale. (I'm prejudiced because I think Airedales and collies are the most intelligent communicating animals.) From personal experience I know that Airedales want to please you and know how to interpret even the slightest human movement. If they feel that you don't understand what they're saying they will often repeat the request again and again.

Sealyham. These lovely, gentle-looking dogs speak often and command a vast vocabulary of barks. They make excellent watchdogs and bark differently when announcing intruders or friends.

Bedlington. This is a very sagacious dog, but is often stubborn and requires a firm but patient owner. Loses interest quickly and it is recommended that two five-minute sessions a day should be sufficient.

Scotch terrier. When the late President Franklin Roosevelt owned Fala, an apocryphal story about him enjoyed great popularity at the time. Fala's cousin, another Scotch terrier, was supposed to have told his owner, a staunch, conservative Republican, "I don't want to have any connection with that horrible man in the White House. From now on refer to me as just a plain terrier!" Not all Scotch terriers possess such vast vocabularies, even in a joke, but most of them want to please their owners. You can anticipate marvelous two-way communication by offering praise, love, and respect.

Mongrels

These dogs vary in size, shape, and in almost every other respect. An animal is referred to as a mongrel when his parents were of mixed breeds. A majority of dogs in the United States belong in this category and many of their owners maintain that "mutts" make superior pets because they are more intelligent. The behaviorists whom I consulted straddled the question and said, "Some are and some are not." They pointed out that among a mongrel's ancestors one might have had some superior ability (such as keen ears) that the mutt inherited. The same might apply to his inheriting some weak characteristic. The owner has to evaluate each case separately. While the dog is achieving his full growth the owner experiences a canine grab bag, never knowing what's going to come out. Few of the numerous breeds we see today are used for any of their original purposes, but most of the animal behaviorists I talked to said that two-way communication requires an owner to be aware of the dog's background.

I was told, *"Don't try to turn the dog into something he was never intended to be!"*

Matthew Margolis, the founder of the National Institute of Dog Training, says, "The owner should try to remember that a Siberian husky shouldn't be switched into a lady's boudoir pet or a Chihuahua into a ferocious guard dog." Margolis, who has successfully trained more than 7500 dogs, added, "I know that sounds facetious, but I've seen uninformed dog owners commit . . . atrocious acts!"

"The man and woman who take time out to observe, understand, and converse with the dog—as he is—can look forward to years of pleasurable and meaningful companionship," says Dr. Borgese. "Such a joint project will benefit both the owner and the animal."

Dr. Borgese has provided a great deal of significant information to human–pet communication with a series of her own experiments. One used the talents of a poodle named Peg who constantly conversed with her mistress, Ms. Ines Giordana Corridori, of Brescia, Italy. Peg was rumored to possess an amazing ability to solve intricate problems. The dog used letter-bearing cards to compose words. She'd pick out a letter with her snout. It sounded so intriguing that Dr. Borgese decided to investigate.

To make certain that there would be no cheating, Dr.

Borgese devised a test that eliminated all chances of collusion. She would arrive at the Corridori residence with her test materials safely locked in a briefcase. She was very careful to make certain that the contents remained secret and she sent Ms. Corridori to the rear of the room, where she was required to turn her back to the dog.

Only then did Dr. Borgese take out the contents of the briefcase—a children's book consisting of large illustrations of domestic animals. She opened the book at random and showed it to the dog, but held it in such a fashion that she herself couldn't see the contents. Nobody could possibly examine the book except Peg, the dog.

After several seconds Dr. Borgese closed the book, returned it to the briefcase, and securely locked it. She then asked the dog to write out what she had seen. Peg promptly used her nose to spell out *cavalli* (horses). Dr. Borgese reopened the briefcase, removed the book, and opened to the place where she had left a mark between the pages. Peg had solved the problem accurately— there was indeed a picture of two large work horses. Peg had not only identified the animals correctly; she had also used the plural, *cavalli*, instead of the singular, *cavallo*.

Dr. Borgese repeated the controlled experiment several times in her own home, making certain that no hidden mirrors had been brought in. The results were the same. Peg correctly spelled out *cane* (dog) and *mucca* (cow). Other animal behaviorists offered all sorts of explanations for the dog's precise performance, and even the most extreme pragmatist agreed that Peg was basically an extraordinarily intelligent animal.

Peg died in August, 1963, and, about that time, Dr. Borgese decided to work with Arli, her own English setter. Dr. Borgese devised a typewriter with keys large enough so Arli could push them down with his nose. In two years of training he learned seventeen letters and could use them to compose more than sixty words. Occasionally the dog felt particularly creative and composed nonsensical free-wheeling poetry.

Currently, Dr. Borgese is in the midst of another fabulous dog communication experiment. While lecturing at the University of California, she is training three dogs in music appreciation. Dr. Borgese starts by singing a note. The dogs then go to a specially built electric organ and pick out the note with their noses. By now they can single out two or more musical notes at a time and hold them for four beats. Dr. Borgese beams at the happy dogs and rewards them with small pieces of raw meat.

Animal behaviorists have discovered that the single most important trait that makes the dog unique is his sincere desire to please and delight humans. Nothing makes him happier than to be told that he is performing up to the owner's expectations—whether this means acting as a seeing-eye dog, a sheepdog, a watchdog, or even as a satisfying household pet. Thus scientists have learned that training is not a question of discipline, but of communication, of letting the dog know exactly what you want him to accomplish. They are discovering that although dogs differ vastly, there are some basic similarities and that the wise owner knows what they are. Here are three familiar types found within every breed:

1. **The "Self-Right" Dog.** Trainers use that term to describe the "ideal" animal. He's self-assured, outgoing, and friendly. However, he has a strong sense of his own rights and his own dignity. He'll greet guests with a wag of his tail, but he has too much dignity to jump on them. He's the easiest dog to converse with, because the owner doesn't have to change undesirable personality traits. He makes the best student and you could start right now teaching him how to converse. Most dogs fall within this category.

2. **The Frightened Dog.** He bites occasionally, not because he's vicious but out of fear and insecurity. Often, the apprehension is the direct result of the owner's insecurity or lack of attention. The owner rarely talks to the dog. When he does, he is likely just to shout "No!" It is possible to break the pattern by being gentle with the dog and teaching him that he has nothing to fear from you. Do this *before* you start your communication sessions.

3. **The Nuisance.** This dog always demands the center of the stage and the owner usually allows him to occupy it. The nuisance dog is basically a decent animal but his owner, often without realizing it, encourages him to jump on guests, to take scraps off the table, and to ignore commands. A newly informed owner can effectively curb the dog's ebullience by letting him know who is boss. This, too, needs your immediate

attention before communication talents can be successfully developed.

There are literally hundreds of books that concern the training of dogs. Many are very informative and will help you solve a special obedience problem, although none deals specifically with communications training. In the preparation of this book I read many of these manuals. The one that intrigued me the most was devoted to dogs and their horoscopes. The book warns the owner that every dog, regardless of breed, needs a yearly anniversary, because birthdays reveal a great deal about the animal. For example, the *Libra* male dog doesn't fall in love forever and is destined to remain fickle in matters of the heart. Despite the large, expressive eyes of *Gemini* dogs, they always make tracks all over your newly waxed kitchen floor.

I suppose horoscopes are useful and may help avoid scuffed floors. The more scientific methods may take a bit longer, but should get more reliable results.

CHAPTER IV

Successful Dog Owners Explain How They Communicate with Their Pets

"One of the main reasons why the dog can be such a close companion to man," says Dr. Fox, the veterinarian, "is because the dog has a very clear language, very similar to ours, that anyone can soon learn to read."

The most ardent believers of this statement are people who have lived with dogs for years. In fact, many of them told me that they don't think that Dr. Fox has gone far enough. A typical comment came from Nancy Lehrman, a laboratory technician in Charlotte, North Carolina.

"Not only can *I* read what the dog says to me," she explained, "but *he* understands what *I* say to him. The proof is that we carry on two-way conversations all the time. Oh, I don't mean discuss philosophy or the high cost of living, but we do talk about the kind of a day we've had or if my neighbor is a gossip—things like that."

I heard similar reports over and over again and the people who uttered them are not quacks, cranks or self-deluders, but highly respected members of their communities. They serve on school boards, church vestries, town councils, hold down responsible positions in business and in the professions, and belong to distinguished organizations. Many can be classified as cautious and conservative—yet when it comes to the subject of their dogs they are far from reticent.

All of them have learned to communicate with their pets. Some of their comments might sound repetitive, but while these dog owners may achieve similar results they often arrive at them via different routes. I feel that you should be offered a wide selection of methods, so *repetition should prove helpful.* Therefore, I suggest that you read the following chapters with extra care! I believe that you will benefit by drawing on the experience of these men and women.

The Doubting Banker

I purposely begin this section with Philip C. Chapman, Jr., because he is without doubt the most pragmatic person I have ever met. In the course of my writing career, I've talked to dozens of men and women whom I labeled "extreme doubters" because of their inherent ultra-suspicious natures. Compared to Chapman, they were just a bunch of Naive Nellies. Not only did Chapman ask for my press credentials; he actually checked them meticulously. Every answer he gave me was care-fully thought out. He has a tendency to pause frequently within his sentences and he told me, "Before I accepted the fact . . . that you can communicate with a dog . . . I had to be mighty certain I wasn't buying a bag of tricks. It becomes second nature not to take anything for granted!"

Chapman is fifty-nine years old, lives in a twelve-room house near Boston, and is considered by his as-sociates to be "a guy who made it big." He is ruggedly handsome, tall and, although thin, appears to be in excellent shape. Despite his craggy good looks he tells you that he has become accustomed to being physically likened to Abraham Lincoln. He chuckles as he says, "I don't have the beard, but everything else fits. . . . Old Abe was ugly, too." He may not really agree with the comparison, but obviously he relishes telling the story.

Chapman has been married for twenty-seven years to his wife, Christina, whose parents were born in Sweden. "It took my mother and father a long time to get over that fact," he said. "When they finally did they told Christina that she was really as good as a lot of 'true-blooded Yankees.' Christina and I still laugh about it."

The Chapmans have three married children who live in other parts of the country. The Chapmans neverthe-less retain the large house because, as Chapman ex-plained, "when they and their spouses come visiting with all their children—we've got eleven grandchil-dren—the house starts leaping!" (Several minutes later Chapman proved his concern over accuracy when he said, "I wasn't completely, categorically honest when I told you about eleven grandchildren. My daughter, El-

len, expects a child sometime this month. The doctor tells her to expect twins, but I won't believe it until I see them. You know, the chances of bearing twins are 1 in 87, and triplets 1 in 7,569. But multiple births in dogs are commonplace. As a matter of fact, when the litter consists of only one puppy there may be cause for alarm, although I have some grave doubts on that score."

Nine years ago Chapman's wife gave him a Kerry blue terrier that he named Casey. The dog sleeps at the foot of his master's bed in an elegant wicker basket lined with authentic Scottish plaid quilting. "I wouldn't invest in such nonsense," he said, "but my son and daughter-in-law gave it to me one Christmas. It's so inordinately extravagant that Casey could use it for collateral on a loan. Come to think of it, I'll wager that he knows the word loan . . . he hears it so often."

Chapman experimented by using the word several times. His voice suddenly became slightly higher pitched. I felt that the dog understood, but it wasn't good enough for Chapman, who said that he'd work on it after I left.

The interview took place in the Chapman library with its four comfortable red leather chairs, a fireplace and hundreds of leather-bound books that look as if they have been read.

Philip C. Chapman, Jr.: "I got Casey because of a heart attack. Those things seem to happen for no apparent reason. No, that isn't quite correct—in my case it occurred because I was pushing myself too hard. You hear about bankers' hours ending at 3 o'clock—that's a laugh—some days I worked until 8 P.M. or later. Often I'd have to go directly from the bank to some community meeting. I hadn't had a real vacation in fifteen years. Whatever the reason, I suffered a severe coronary and was hospitalized for three weeks and had to take it easy for many weeks afterward. That's when Christina presented me with Casey. She thought that a dog would be good for me.

"I'd never owned a dog before, although I did have some hamsters and white mice. Once my sister Julia tried to bring a stray mongrel into our house, but my father had a fit. He said that dogs were carriers of disease and that was that. In those days fathers still ruled the roost! He died years ago, but I'm sure he'd still want me to keep the 'junior' after my name. I hope my son does the same, but I doubt it.

"You can't resist a young puppy for very long. Casey was eleven weeks when Christina brought him and he looked like a tiny fur muff that an Eskimo child might wear. Don't you believe that a banker's heart is cold as steel. Inside of a week, I found myself talking to Casey—not baby talk, but simple sentences I might use with my grandchildren. He seemed to respond best when I raised my voice higher than usual—sort of a semi-high pitch. . . . To make sure that he really comprehended what I was saying, I'd speak contrary words in an ordinary tone.

"Instead of saying, 'Let's go out,' I'd tell him something far-fetched like, 'Now is the time for all good men to come to the aid of their party.' He didn't respond. I reasoned that this was because the sentence contained so many additional words. So I said, 'Don't be mad.' Still no response. He'd look at me quizzically, as if to say, 'What are you talking about?' Then I'd say, in the higher voice, 'Let's go out.' He'd quickly fetch the leash!

"I'd repeat words over and over; use them in short sentences. For example, the word might be *door* and I'd start by saying, 'Door, door, door.' Then I'd show him a door in one of the bedrooms. This time I'd say, 'Here is a bedroom *door.*' The emphasis would be on *door.* I'd do the same thing in other rooms and before long he'd recognize the word. That was the time for a reward. He likes Oreo crackers and I'd give him one with an accompanying pat. I'd always add something like, 'You're a very smart dog!'

"I also discovered that he had a very short learning span and I'd get best results if I didn't work with him for too long a time. Our eventual routine was ten minutes in the morning before I left for the bank and again for ten minutes just after dinner—both his and mine. I've learned that it's difficult to glean knowledge on an empty stomach.

"His vocabulary increased and I'll hazard a guess that it's now ... well over a hundred. Dr. William J. Funk, the noted lexicographer, claimed that the average dog has a vocabulary of about 60 words and an exceptional dog could comprehend 250 words. I'd rate Casey somewhere in between.

"Understanding him presented a more difficult problem. I realized that he was saying things, but I just couldn't fathom what he was telling me. Then I started to think ... he could understand me ... did that mean

52

that he was the more intelligent and I the inferior? That seemed to go in the face of all scientific study . . . at the very least I was equally as bright. That was when I decided to observe him carefully. I'd always looked at him, naturally, but I honestly can't say how carefully. Now I watched his every move, every grimace, every expression.

"I watched very vigilantly . . . and very often. I'd notice that he constantly used the same movement or expression for a specific action. It got so that I knew that when his ears were cocked, his face tilted to the left, and when he issued several short, clipped barks, he was saying, **'I am in total agreement.'** Ears down, face tilted to the right side, and a short series of high-pitched barks meant, **'No, I don't agree.'**

"Tail wagging while he's in a crouch and when nudging me with his snout means, **'I think we ought to try that.'** When he sticks his tongue in and out and beams at me, he's saying, **'I'm your pal forever.'** When he suddenly squeals with delight and his ears and tail go up, he's telling me, **'Christina's car has just come up the driveway.'** Many, many things of that sort.

"My advice to dog owners . . . who want to understand . . . their pets . . . is: *'Observe, and ye shall reap!'* "

"The Most Intelligent Member of the Family"

Melida Marver was half-joking, half-serious when she offered me the above description of Antoine, her nine-year-old French poodle. Melida modestly refuses to take full credit for the amazing animal, but it's very apparent that she is chiefly responsible for the dog's being able to communicate so well with humans.

I met Melida and John Marver at the Richmond, Virginia, airport where they had come to meet my plane. I had heard lavish tales about this astonishing dog and I had come to see for myself. The Marvers are the parents of two young children, Jennifer and Robert, and live in an elegant, large brick house in Richmond, where Mr. Marver is the manager of radio station WANT.

"At first I wanted to strangle that dog," Mr. Marver told me. "I was courting Melida at the time and I told her that I was thirty-three years old. One evening we were watching the dog perform one of his outstanding feats—he was supposed to guess your age by barking the appropriate number of years. My turn came and I wrote 'thirty-three' on a piece of paper. Antoine started barking and didn't stop at thirty-three, but continued on to thirty-six. Melida apologized for his rudeness and ordered him to re-do it. Antoine repeated, again not stopping until he reached thirty-six. Melida said, 'Antoine, you goofed twice,' and the chastised dog slunk off. Later that evening I confessed that I was really thirty-six. Now, I don't think that Antoine is some uncanny mind reader, but it's certainly evident that he is highly intelligent and that my wife has made excellent use of that intelligence. The dog must have sensed that I was tense when he came to thirty-three and unconsciously I probably did something when he reached thirty-six—it could have been a tiny movement of the eyes or the hands—even a change of expression. No matter what, from that day on, I no longer took Antoine for granted."

Melida Marver is slender, dark-haired, exceptionally

pretty, and very, very busy. The phone rang constantly and in a charming Southern accent she turned down invitations to tea, a club meeting, and a bridge luncheon. She said that she was sorry to refuse, but couldn't make it because of a visitor; because she had agreed to play tennis that afternoon; because she would be collecting clothes for the needy; and because she had promised to take her children to a puppet show.

We sat in the Marver den, which is tastefully decorated in a soft green and has many subsidiary pieces; among them were several large hanging plants, pictures of the children, and a modern sculpture of the Madonna and child. I was told that Antoine enjoys looking at pretty things. About two hours later, Ruth, the family maid, told us that lunch was ready. Melida asked Antoine if he would like some lunch. He barked his assent and followed us into the kitchen, where he was given hamburger meat. When he finished, he barked again. Melida explained those additional barks: "He says, 'Please, may I have some more?'"

Melida Marver: "I got Antoine's name from a beauty parlor I used to go to. It seemed so suitable—he really is a handsome animal. Don't you agree? Those ribbons on his ears look so nice. Oh, drat, one of them must have fallen off. That's why he barked before, he was telling me about it, but I was busy in the kitchen at the time and didn't listen.

"At first Antoine couldn't bark at all; he'd whine instead. I was worried and tried to teach him by getting down on all fours and barking like I thought a dog

55

should. I remember one day the doctor came to treat some other member of the family and saw my strange performance. He must have thought I had suddenly gone berserk. He told my mother that perhaps she should consult a psychiatrist about me.

"Eventually, Antoine got his bark and has been barking since. Perhaps my crawling on hands and knees helped. An owner should remember that the dog has to look up and see the world—most everything must seem pretty big to him!

"After he learned how to bark I would point a finger at him. One finger elicited one bark, two fingers two barks, and so forth. Every time he did it I'd praise his performance and give him a reward. Antoine, like most dogs, has definite likes and dislikes. There was no point in offering him a reward that he didn't like. As a matter of fact, sometimes a bad reward had an adverse effect. I knew he liked cheese and bits of hot dogs; so that is what I gave him.

"One day a very good friend of mine came visiting and I wanted to show her how smart Antoine was. I held up fingers and Antoine barked accordingly. That made me all aglow and I was carried away. I said he could even do math problems. Then I asked Antoine what one and one were. I was going to put two fingers behind my friend's back, but before I could do it Antoine barked twice. Quickly, I tried two and two. Four barks. After that triumph Antoine and I practiced far into the night, but he soon got tired and his performance fell off. That's always the case.

"You'll say that I solve problems in my head for him, but you have to admit that, if that's the case, Antoine is smart enough to pick up the appropriate clues. Whatever the reason is, it worked. Then I started telling him simple things like, 'Don't lie on the couch.' He seemed to understand. I drew up easy rules but not very many —an abundance of rules only tends to confuse the dog and nothing is accomplished.

"When Antoine disobeyed I'd make him sit in the corner. That didn't happen very often, but he knew that he was being punished. After a while he'd start barking; he'd be saying, **'I'll be good from now on. May I come out?'**

"Next I worked out a simple system: Antoine would bark once for **'yes,'** twice for **'no,'** and three times for **'I don't know.'** It took some time for him to master the system, but, when he did, it opened up vast new horizons. I was actually able to converse with him and it wasn't difficult. It got so I didn't have to face him to get results. Many times I'd be in the kitchen and I'd ask him if someone was at the door or if the children had come home. That one-two-three barking saved me many, many steps.

"My husband regards Antoine as a pet. I'll have to be honest and admit that to me he is more like a child, but then I regard all pets as children. But I don't humanize Antoine to the extent of taking him to the picture show or making him wear boots when it rains. I do believe that treating him like a member of the family pays off—it helps me know what he's thinking. That isn't as difficult as you'd think; a dog wants his immediate needs attended to, he wants to be fed, to be loved, to be kept in good health.

"Once Antoine had a sore throat and he started to

bark and raise his paw upward, almost pointing to his throat. That didn't require any special supernatural gift on my part—it was so obvious. I asked him, 'Do you have a sore throat?' He barked once and his face showed the pain, so I took him to the vet. But then it was some of the same when Jennifer and Bob were tiny infants; their cries would often tell me whey they were ailing. I've learned to be attentive to Antoine's signals in the same way. Just think how much easier it would be for an owner if she knew when her dog was asking for a drink of water—and also easier for the dog!

"I suppose there are some drawbacks to my making him one of the family. His birthday is on June twenty-fifth and he always receives a stuffed toy for a present. He will play with it until a week before his birthday and then rip it to shreds in preparation for his new stuffed toy. It's funny to see a dog go up to bed with a stuffed rabbit in his mouth. He won't go to sleep without it and sometimes he whines when he forgets it.

"Also, when we have a birthday party he insists on being part of the group. He loves festive occasions and eats birthday cake and ice cream—extra-large portions. He doesn't like sweets on other occasions.

"I sometimes wonder why Antoine is so superior. You don't really suppose it's because his food used to be spiced with garlic? I once read that garlic was brain food and took it seriously; I'd give him large doses. That is until the neighbors started to complain about the aroma!"

"It's Far Better to Receive"

Leon Wolfer was born in Boston, but has lived on Manhattan's West Side for many years. He knows—and likes—most of the dogs in a three-block radius from his home. And they know—and like—him. He is a bachelor and feels that for a person living alone a dog makes an ideal companion. "They are a tremendous help in avoiding loneliness," he says. "When you learn to carry on conversations with your dog you no longer have the need to talk to yourself."

Wolfer is a salesman in a stationery store near his house and keeps a section of one of the counters filled with dog biscuits. "Whenever a dog comes in I give him a biscuit and he promptly thanks me," Wolfer says. "Do me something—I like dogs." He walks them and takes care of them when their owners are away. As a result he has some very definite thoughts and one of his strong opinions concerns purebreds versus mongrels. Wolfer prefers the latter.

"Most of the dogs I have owned," he says, "were mixed breeds. They seem to be more intelligent. Purebreds inherit both the best and the worst. It's often just a pure case of snobbery to say that your basset hound was fathered by Lancelot V and is the third cousin of Champion Lady Godiva IX."

Wolfer is a short, middle-aged man and possesses a keen sense of humor. He believes that dogs also have a sense of humor. "They must," he says. "Why else would my Lassie laugh at my jokes?"

To get more information about Wolfer I spoke to other

dog owners in his neighborhood. They were unanimous in singing his praise. One of them told me, "Dogs know who their true friends are, and not only does my collie jump for joy when he sees Leon, but he starts talking to him. You should see the two of them carry on! Leon's a man who believes that, where dogs are concerned, it's far better to receive."

Leon Wolfer: "It depends on the owner how fast the dog learns to communicate. In my case I took my Lassie home and we started right off 'talking' to each other. I told her that if she was a good girl and got along with my other dog—they were both called Lassie and to distinguish them I added numbers I and II—she would be taken care of. I said all this in a firm but gentle tone and I also did a lot of gesturing. I felt that she understood what I was saying when she walked over to Lassie I and actually kissed her—I swear she did. Then she wagged her tail and looked straight at me as if to say, **'Okay, it's a deal!'** From that day on Lassie I and II got on well.

"If she did something wrong, like ripping up a pillow, I'd take the end of the leash and tap her gently. Some trainers don't approve of doing that, but personally I find that it works. Then I'd say, 'Stay in the bedroom.' She'd slink off into the bedroom, but like a naughty child she'd soon come out. She'd pout like some of the kids I see in the store when their mothers refuse to buy them a lollipop or a chocolate bar. I'd make her go back, because I believe that consistency is very important. I can count on one hand the number of times I have had to punish Lassie, but I've learned that it helps tremendously to follow through and show your displeasure. You have to play the punishment bit by ear. Lassie was cowed when I got her and I felt that punishment would make her even more upset and high strung.

"On my way to work in the morning, I'd see a dog staring out of a ground floor window—she looked so forlorn. I guessed she was part springer spaniel and part poodle. One warm day the window was open and I stopped and patted her; she seemed so grateful. From that day on, I always had to stop to greet her; she seemed to expect it.

"Lassie was part of a large litter—seventeen puppies. She was the runt and, although the owner had found homes for all the others, no one wanted to take her. It was about six years ago and I had Lassie I at the time; I didn't have the slightest intention of owning another animal. Then a family who lived in my house had their dog stolen and their little boy was heartbroken. I thought they'd be happy if I got that dog for them, so I did, and they asked me to keep her for a short while until they moved.

"They were in the process of buying a house in Tappan, New York, and had run into a tax problem. By the time they got clear title six months later, I'd grown very fond of the dog. That's when I learned that Lassie I had to be put to sleep. Fortunately, the family that I had intended to give her to had acquired another dog and they weren't very upset when I told them I wanted to keep Lassie II.

"Now I found myself talking to her all the time. I

61

suppose some people will say I'm nuts, but I advise dog owners not to care about what anyone says and *keep on talking!* Oh, I don't mean 'itsy-bitsy' palaver or puffing on a long cigar while you're both discussing the stock market. But tell the dog about your sister's health or about the conversation you just had on the telephone. Remember, the more extensive and frequent the conversations, the more the dog will understand. It's as simple as that.

"Let's say that tonight I'll look at television. Lassie would be surprised and might butt into the TV set and then bark sharply at it. A few seconds later she'd do the same thing to me. From experience, I'd know that she was saying, **'What in the hell are you doing? You don't watch TV at night.'** Then I begin to explain about it being a special show. You might think all this is screwy, but I've found that although the dog may not understand the exact words, she gets some idea of what I'm saying.

"In teaching her I use short sentences, but seldom just one word. I'm a firm believer that short, crisp commands are so very impersonal. When you just say, 'sit,' 'stay,' 'jump,' they're too cold for my taste. Instead, I tell her, 'Lassie, I want you to come. That's a good girl.'

"I must say in all honesty that I think she's probably responding to the key word, 'come,' but I feel she is far happier when I'm more conversational. And comprehension grows. For example, when I tell her, 'Take a pill, it'll make you feel better,' she does. The first time I said that to her she didn't know what in the world I was referring to. Now when she hears the word 'pill' she might make a long face, but she opens her mouth.

"I believe it's best to work with your dog after she's gone out for a brisk walk. Let's face it, you can't learn very well when you have to urinate or move your bowels. I also discovered that I wasn't the best teacher when I was tired. If I had an especially hard day, I'd postpone the lesson until the following evening. Another thing I found is: don't rush your animal. Give her plenty of time to show you what she's trying to say. It may take a lot of time, but I believe it's worth it. I'm sure that Lassie cooperates because she wants to please me. She likes to be told how clever she is. Most dogs do.

"One of the games that people often play is charades—it's even a leading television show. If human beings can be made to interpret your silent language, why can't dogs?"

A Legal Approach to Dog Communication

No one sounds more knowledgeable about the law than a law student, and Alice Milmed Haller isn't any exception. She is in her second year of law school and is about to take her exams; if her excellent scholastic record is any indication of her legal acumen she should breeze right through them. She comes from a legal family: her father is a judge and her brother is completing law school.

"Only my mother isn't identified with the law," Alice said, almost apologetically. "She's a college philosophy professor. But I'm quite sure that she could deliver an erudite lecture about Socrates and the early law!"

Although Alice is more gregarious than her husband, Mike, they both are attractive, sensitive, intelligent people and obviously very much in love. I don't know if Alice Haller can prepare a chocolate soufflé, but I get the feeling that she would prefer doing that than darning her husband's socks.

Mike is a musician and a carpenter; he would like to combine careers by designing and building musical studios and recital halls and testing some theories he has about proper acoustics.

"Our dog, Sam, should be very helpful," he told me. "Did you know that a dog's hearing is vastly superior to man's and that the dog can detect high frequencies that the human ear cannot?"

Last year the Hallers became the owners of an Airedale puppy they named Sam. The trio—Alice, Mike and Sam—live in San Francisco and while the (human) Hallers constantly praise that fabulous city— verbally—Sam is a booster in his own way. He opens his eyes wide, wags his tail, flicks his ears, and emits a series of joyous barks. I was told that he is saying, "San Francisco, I'm glad you opened your Golden Gates for me!"

Alice Haller: "The other day Mike saw another Airedale who reminded him of Sam. The Airedale had a leash hanging free and had just obviously gotten out of a car. He was standing there with his face forward, ears back—eagerly waiting for instructions—just like Sam. If the owner delivers them in a clear, precise fashion, the dog will most likely follow through, Sam tries to.

"When we got him he had another name—King. It

was much too fancy and we didn't feel that it was very appropriate. We wanted something real simple; when we listened to the Watergate hearings, I fell in love with Senator Sam Ervin from North Carolina—I guess something good came out of Watergate after all; it provided the name. Like his namesake, Sam is very gentle, yet persuasive. He isn't insistent on being fed, but he loves to go out and urges me to take him in my car. He knows that when I do we will wind up in the park and then he can have a long walk. He usually does it on Saturday and Sunday, when I'm home and not at school.

"I've discovered that dogs do best when they have decided rituals—they like to do things at the same time every day. In the morning Sam puts his feet up on our bed, and he expects us to pet him a little. Then he waits patiently while Mike and I wash. He listens to the news with us. Mike takes him to work with him and Sam always goes in advance down the stairs. Little things, but they mean a lot to a dog.

"From the start, Mike and I decided to give Sam free run of the house—that is: everything but my study. For some reason, I'm uptight about it. But Sam seems to be unaware of that room and appears to be perfectly happy. I guess a happy dog makes for good communication. There are other aids that we have discovered:

• "The earlier I detected a problem the easier I found it to cure. But often it required a great deal of will power."

• "We always smile at Sam and let him know how much we like him."

- "We don't give in to his every fancy. There are times when we have to stand firm. That's hard to do, but it pays off."

- "We let him know that we aren't afraid of him. This may sound silly, but I've seen a lot of owners who actually fear their dogs."

- "Mike and I offer a lot of patience, but not unlimited patience."

- "We speak up. We learned that if you're always silent when you do things for him, he notices the lack of communication and remains in his own shell. Not that I'm frequently very quiet."

- "Sam has learned what he can and cannot do. So have we."

"The last bit of advice I picked up on the long-distance phone. When we first brought Sam home, the very first thing I did was to try to take him out for a walk. We didn't have a leash, so I put a small rope around his neck and started down the steps. He didn't budge, so I started dragging him. Still a negative response. I was furious and almost in tears; I had heard that Airedales were stubborn, but this was too much. I pulled harder, but still he wouldn't stir. Finally, I took the rope off and we remained in the apartment.

"I put in a call to a friend of mine who lives in New York and has owned several Airedales. I told her my tragic tale. She listened intently and then started laughing. 'He's just a tiny puppy,' she finally said. 'Only eight weeks old and you expect him to act grown up. Take it easy!' That was excellent counseling and I pass it on to you because I believe it's essential for good two-way communication.

"We've had dogs ever since I was a child, but my mother had always taken care of them. She knows a great deal about animals and has a marvelous way with them. I remember when Mother came home she'd say to the dog, 'Nellie, it's just me.' Evidently, this greeting long bothered Mother. Recently she told me why. 'It's ungrammatical,' she said, 'but I'd feel silly saying, 'Nellie, it's only I.'

"That's another bit of good advice: Don't look silly to your dog!"

CHAPTER V

More
Dog Owners Explain

Lew + Buddy = Two Buddies

Most pet owners think that their animals are without a doubt the very smartest in the world. Lew Burke is no exception, and in his case there are many who agree with him. Lew is the owner of Buddy, an eight-year-old black German shepherd who constantly astounds audiences with his performances. Lew and Buddy have appeared on more than forty national television shows. Among them: "Johnny Carson," "Merv Griffin," "Mike Douglas," "To Tell the Truth," "Soupy Sales," "Wonderama," "Captain Kangaroo." The pair are usually summoned back for repeat performances and they change the act. Though their routine may vary, one thing remains constant—the close communication that exists between Lew and Buddy.

Lew Burke is only in his late thirties but he has a very checkered past. When he graduated from college, where he received both a B.S. and a Master's degree, he went on to dental school, but the thought of pulling teeth didn't appear to be very exciting so he decided to box professionally. (Earlier he had fought as an amateur in the Golden Gloves, where he won twenty-one fights and went on to the finals.) Lew was an immediate success in the lightweight division, knocking out five straight opponents. Sportswriters called him "a definite comer and possible champion." But Lew became restless again and started teaching health education and physical training. By accident, he discovered his true vocation—animal trainer and entertainer.

Buddy has had an equally full career. He was given away at the age of thirteen months by his first owner, who thought he was too retarded to keep; he had flunked out of obedience school. Lew took the maligned and frightened dog and six months later he appeared with him on "The Johnny Carson Show," where he showed his virtuosity by adding, subtracting, and multiplying. Buddy successfully solved all of Carson's mathematical problems by selecting the correct answers from a circle of numbers. "Granted," says Burke, "it was a trick, but the dog was clever enough to master it!"

Meanwhile, Buddy had endeared himself to Lew's four children and all the other youngsters in the neighborhood. He even rescued one from a burning building. Buddy has made many movies; his most recent one was For Pete's Sake, *starring Barbra Streisand. The dog was on the screen for ten minutes and in one complicated chase scene—for which he had to learn his part right on the set—Barbra Streisand was so impressed that she said to Lew, "It's sheer magic the way you and Buddy talk to each other!"*

Lew's reply was, "Anyone can learn how."
I talked to Lew and Buddy in their animal training clinic in Brooklyn. Occasionally, the barking of other dogs interrupted our conversation. They didn't appear to be angry barks—just appropriate background sounds.

Lew Burke: "Communication between dogs and humans exists! I'm positive of that fact! Every day of the week, I talk to Buddy and he talks to me. Granted, I'm probably prejudiced by thinking Buddy is cleverer than all other dogs, but after training dogs for fifteen years I'm certain that anyone can succeed in chatting with a dog. I've discovered three things have to be present if you desire good communication:

"1. *Love.* That old saying, 'Love me, love my dog' should be changed to '*love your dog.*' A dog is an excellent judge of *Homo sapiens* and can easily spot a phony—someone who pretends to love, but to whom love is just a sham.

"2. *Respect.* You have to realize that respect and love are not the same thing—you need to have both! An owner should be aware that dogs have certain inalienable rights. They may not be defined in the Declaration of Independence, but they exist. Many people only pretend that they feel very tender toward their dogs and would swear they respect them. Nonsense!

"3. *Patience.* I'm lucky that Buddy is a quick study. Your dog might not learn so fast, but that doesn't mean that you have to throw up your hands in surrender. By training all varieties of dogs, I've found that some dogs require things explained to them over and over and over, so I do it; it requires a little more time, but very little else. Remember, all dogs, like human beings, are different. Studying your dog will reveal his temperament.

"You've probably seen or read about wild dog packs. Well, all those packs have a leader—someone definitely in charge. When the dog is in so-called civilized society, we domesticate him, but the dog still wants someone to assume that leadership role. Unlike the cat, who is an independent animal, he urgently needs someone to be in charge.

"His number one choice is you—he wants you, the owner, to assume that role. If you abdicate, then you can expect to have a very mixed-up dog. He wants you to be strong. That means that when you ask him to do something—within reason—he should do it. *You're not the dog's leader if you don't!*

"This doesn't mean that you should become a Simon Legree and treat him like a slave. Where he's concerned, moderation is the proper role. If you're not sure how you should behave, a good rule of thumb to follow is 'Would I like that done to me?' If the answer is 'no' then you should probably desist.

"One thing that contributes to good communication is to sometimes feed the dog by hand. That is one of the ways to let him know you are his friend. Bear in mind that dogs don't reason the way human beings do. To them, black is black and white is white—no in-betweens. Therefore, the hand should only offer friendship—never punishment! When you use the hand for both, the dog becomes confused. Fortunately, I don't have to punish Buddy. If I did I would never, never do it with my hand!

"See how Buddy is aware of the whole situation. He hears his name mentioned, and even though he seems to be resting, his ears are up and he's listening to our conversation. If I made a sudden move, he'd be right there. Most dogs are that way—they know a great deal more than we credit them with. I'll bet the owner of the average dog could be sitting in a comfortable chair and suddenly raise his arm or his voice. Immediately, he'd see the dog's ears go up and the dog would probably come to investigate. I suggest you try it on your dog—try it right now.

"The owner should constantly realize that his dog is observant. He sees—and knows—a lot more than you think he does. If I take my shoes and socks off, Buddy knows I'm not planning to go out. He walks to the side of my chair and lies down. That's when *I know that he knows* what my intentions are.

"There should be a test for dog ownership. Questions like: *How do you react when a dog 'misbehaves' and defecates?* After all, it's a very natural function—and if a would-be owner is totally repulsed by the smell he shouldn't own a dog. You're taking a living thing into your home, not a machine.

"Another question might be: *Do you shudder when he sheds or jumps on furniture?* If that's the case, I'd advise you to buy a stuffed animal. The owner who wants a dog who barks at possible intruders at the door, but never at people in normal situations, should get a tape recording of a bark—I hear they're now available. Or, if you want a dog who shows affection, who loves you, but never touches his tongue to your face, get a . . . I don't know what to suggest. We have to be honest with ourselves when we acquire or possess an animal—do we really want it?

"You might ask me what does all this have to do with communication? A great deal! You'll be able to carry on conversations with your dog only if you honestly and truly want the dog. The next thing you might say is that some people have a natural way with animals, like possessing a green thumb for gardening—either you have it or you don't. My daughter, Elizabeth, has that quality. She talks to animals all the time. She'll be practicing on the piano and a pet bird that lives with us will perch on her shoulder; he won't do that with any other member of the family.

"Sure, that quality is great, but all it means is that people who don't possess it have to work a little harder—I do believe it can be acquired. And when you do, you'll be a happier person—and your dog will be happier, too. You have to remember that there are many similarities. When you encounter a locked door you may start yelling to attract attention. Well, the dog does pretty much the same thing by barking."

The Story Book Family

Several years ago there was a children's book about a family named Sanders who lived on a farm, had lots of animals, a shiny red tractor, and had built a house with their very own hands. The author may not have known it, but there actually is such a family; you only have to add a "u" to the name.

Flip and Sandy Saunders and their two young children, Kate and Andy, live on a farm in Garrison, New York. Like the Sanderses, they also built a house with their very own hands, ride around on a shiny red tractor, and have lots of animals. Among them is a nine-year-old setter named Turk.

Turk has been with the Saunders since he was a tiny puppy. "He's a full-fledged member of the family," says the mother. The children agree and eight-year-old Kate explains, "When we go on a hay wagon ride, Turk always wants to come along. That's only fair since he knows he's one of us."

Sandy is the co-owner of a metal casting firm, but devotes all his free time to operating the 160-acre farm. The farm is no rich man's tax dodge. Sandy works long hours running it. He tends the cows, sheep, and horses, tills the fields, and is in the process of putting a new roof on the barn. The children take care of the chickens. Flip helps run the farm when she isn't performing her duties as a public health nurse. Her medical training has undoubtedly played an important role in making her an ideal animal owner.

I talked to the Saunders family in their large country kitchen that had the appearance of a Currier and Ives lithograph. There was a heaping platter of homemade corn muffins that Flip had just baked. Several pairs of mittens hung on a rope that was attached to the stove, and below them stood four pairs of rubber boots.

Flip Saunders: "Taking care of a dog is very much like taking care of a child—many of the same guidelines apply. I used them on Turk, and that may be why we're able to converse with him. Not long ago, I had occasion to put my theory to a test. I was out with the children and when we got back to the house we discovered fresh blood on the front steps. Turk usually was present to greet us, but this time he wasn't around and we promptly knew he was in trouble. We called and called, but he didn't respond. Finally, we found him. He was covered with blood. I could see that his eye had been seriously injured and knew that I should take him immediately to the vet.

"I told Turk to stay put until I went back to the house to fetch a blanket. I assured him I'd be right back and then we'd go to the vet. I could see Turk understood me; he barked weakly and his facial expression clearly indicated his thoughts. He was saying, **'I was in a fight with another dog and I'm sorry to cause you all this trouble. I'll wait right here.'**

"I had a broken arm at the time, but with the children's help I managed to get Turk into the car and get him to the vet. In a few months we were delighted to see that Turk was almost as good as new—but the fight had cost him an eye.

"There are so many parallels in raising dogs and children. I've talked to some of my pediatrician and veterinarian friends and they tell me the similarity is staggering. Many of the rules apply to two-way communication; if you don't have a healthy animal, you can't expect healthy communication. I suppose animal and child communications boil down to 'need.' If you don't need anything, you don't communicate.

"Saying 'No' constantly to a dog and child often produces the same results—*nothing!* Very often the very first thing a new owner says to his dog is that negative command. It may be because there's a lot of bric-a-brac around the house and the owner is afraid the dog will knock it over. So the owner shouts 'No!' The dog understands, barks slightly, and does just what he's told not to. It's far easier to move the bric-a-brac than to continuously scold. Or the dog may jump on the couch to see how angry you get. Better to remove and distract him than just to say, 'No!'

"The dog often warns you in advance what his intentions are. Learn to interpret them. A good way to do that is by physical contact. Not only does he enjoy being petted, but he'll express himself better if you come closer. Many's the time I've seen people try to discipline their animals almost by remote control—they'd be a dozen feet away.

"The emotional tone also is important. How you say something is often more important than what you say. Turk understands some key words like *barn, car, other house, let's go, horses, tractor.* When we use them in a sentence he picks up the thought by how we enunciate it. We don't say, 'I'm going to feed the horses,' exactly in the same tone as, 'Don't run after that car!'

"I've found that parents are often afraid of their child and that's another thing that applies to a dog: *Don't be scared of him!* He knows when you are and will act accordingly.

"Also, it's easy to get in the habit of misreading his body language. I know some people who think that when their dog starts to wiggle he's about to do something bad. I've observed that Turk starts wiggling when he's happy. I've discovered other Turk 'talk' by looking and listening; when I hear a scratching sound, I know immediately he's locked in somewhere; when he gives a series of short, decisive barks, I know someone is in the driveway; when he opens his mouth slightly, his ears become erect, and he starts growling, I know that he's spotted a woodchuck or some other small animal.

"Turk gets confused when more than one person speaks to him at a time. I've also found that Turk has a conscience. He lets you know when he feels he has done some mischief—his ears go back and he looks guilty. I suppose every dog acts a bit differently, so I'd advise any owner to get to know the dog. I firmly believe that when you get to know and understand your pet you'll also understand yourself better."

"Sheepherding Is Lonely Business, So Thanks for My Dog"

Most of the pet owners I talked to regarded the sheep-herder's job as the most romantic in the world. Not only can the sheepherder avoid the crowded city by being alone on the empty prairie, blanketed by thousands of stars, but he also possesses a very intelligent dog that he can converse with constantly.

Thirty-eight-year-old Miguel Mendez, who has been tending sheep for a long time, has a slightly different description. "Hay qui tomar la vida como si fuera aspirina [*You have to take life like swallowing an aspirin*]," *he said. Miguel quickly added,* "José, my col-

lie dog thinks it makes life 'menos mal [less bad].' "

I met Miguel Mendez in a small hotel-restaurant in San Francisco, where vacationing Basque herders often take their holiday. It was dinnertime and we all ate at a long common table. There were heaping platters of rice, lamb, and cheese. The food was simple but filling. All the sheepherders wore their traditional berets, which they didn't remove during the meal. One also had a bright blue cape that he proudly told me had once belonged to a "muy grande" *bullfighter.*

Although Mendez has been in this country for more than twenty years he still often resorts to Spanish, but speaks English with great dignity, carefully pronouncing each word. It was late fall when I met him and he told me that he was taking his annual holiday. But he had come to San Francisco for another reason, too. "My employer says it is necessary for me to visit this city; he said to see the doctor because for some unknown reason I have a great pain in my chest. Tomorrow, I shall visit the doctor."

Another sheepherder, sitting at the end of the table, laughed. "Miguel," he shouted, "you have been telling us that for a week. You will not visit the doctor tomorrow or the next tomorrow or the next. You will return to your sheep and will die with them." All the others started laughing and soon Miguel joined in. He said something in rapid Spanish that I couldn't interpret. It must have been very funny because the laughter grew louder and the other diners pounded on the table.

When the meal was over Miguel and I moved to the lobby. It badly needed refinishing, but Miguel said, "Has it not great dignity?" We sat in two huge baronial chairs that looked as if they had once belonged in William Randolph Hearst's San Simeon. They, too, needed refinishing, but they were surprisingly comfortable.

Miguel Mendez: "I am in your country because of your very distinguished Senator McCarran. If it was not for that very eminent gentleman, I would still be back in my village in Spain. Did you know that the honorable senator himself once tended sheep? He knew we Basques are excellent herders, so he had us exempted from the quota that applied to all the other Spaniards. And that is why I am here.

"With your kind permission may I drink some more of the wine? It is very good. . . . At the very first I worked in Idaho, but then the son of my father's brother came to California and I followed him.

"In the summer it is most lonely and forsaken. For many months I see no other man but the tender who comes on horseback to bring me supplies. He stays but little since he has many such stops to make. Do not feel that I'm complaining. I have my dog and my radio to keep me company. They both offer much comfort. But if I had to choose between them the choice would indeed be simple—the dog! Not because of the work he does, but for the companionship he offers! The radio is mechanical—not so the dog!

"Some people think that the sheepherder seeks for female company and so services the sheep. It has no truth. It is a very rare thing when such happens. There may have been such happenings, but truly very seldom.

That I would know because we Basques talk to each other when we need and we are very truthful. I have never had such urge—not that I should be sainted.

"Once I possessed two dogs, but my Pedro died of old age and I didn't replace him. José, my present dog, does the work of two animals. He is truly magnificent. I have learned many things from him—but then I have taught him many things, too. If I were told I had to work with another dog I would leave my job at once. José and I are tuned together—we are like one. I talk to him all of the time; he knows that I regard him as the smartest and the best dog around. It is very necessary to make your dog think that. And once you have done that, your dog will do most anything for you. But never tell him falsehoods—he will soon know it if you do.

"At the beginning I taught José simple signs: 'come,' 'good dog,' 'down.' When he was eight weeks old I got a piece of stout rope that was about six feet long and I tied it to his collar. I taught advanced things like 'heel,' and 'stay.' I whirled him around in circles, and when he appeared to be dizzy, I gave the commands again to see if he then would respond. *Never, never give a command that you do not have the desire to see carried out.* I would never tell him to go to the gates of Hell, but if I did I would expect him to carry out my order!

"My commands were always within reason. I'd teach by repeating things over and over. I'd say, *'Bring sheep. Bring sheep.'* At the beginning when I said that José was a disillusionment to me since he would obey my command by bringing me tree branches. But the Virgin Mother was good and José finally learned what I meant by *'bring sheep'* and soon he did the proper thing.

"There is a fine story about bringing in the sheep. I have heard it many times, but I am always delighted to hear it again. It is best told with a glass of wine. With your kind permission may I have another?

"This didn't happen to me, but the Basque herders tell it often. Once there was a herder who was very fond of the whiskey bottle and he would drink in great quantities. One day, it was time to fetch in the sheep and he told his dog, 'Luis, bring in the sheep.' There were one hundred sheep in the flock. Luis brought in ninety-nine. The drunken herder counted them and said in a dirty manner, 'Luis, you are a very bad dog! You only brought in ninety-nine! Get the other one!'

"Luis hung his head and with great shame went off. He looked and looked, but could not find the missing sheep. Finally, in desperation, he jumped over a neighbor's fence and stole a sheep. Triumphantly he brought it to his master. Meantime, the drunken sheepherder had recounted his flock and discovered that indeed he had made a mistake—there were actually the proper number, one hundred!

"I never give José a direct order, but instead tell him, 'You should be guarding the sheep, not sitting under the tree.' José understands and immediately goes there. He is not embarrassed and neither am I. I learned long ago that dogs are very sensitive and deeply resent being called down in front of other dogs or even sheep! When I had Pedro I never scolded him in the presence of José or vice versa. I'd always wait until we were in complete privacy. That is my opinion and I think it is a proper one.

"I never kick the dog. Sometimes I take him by the

neck and gently shake him, but I never abuse or use a whip. When José does what I want him to do I offer him a kind word and a pat on the head. *Gracias a Dios sale bien* [Thanks be to God it always works]."

CHAPTER VI

How Cats Communicate

In ancient Egypt anyone who intentionally killed a cat was put to death. When an Egyptian cat died, members of the household were required by law to shave off their eyebrows as a badge of respect. In one important battle with the Romans, the Egyptians sacrificed an entire city rather than take the risk of killing any of the cats that the enemy had deliberately brought into battle. The Romans knew that Egyptians held the cat sacred and asked three questions of anyone who questioned the animal's worthiness:

"Did not the cat's eyes still shine at night, reflecting the rays of the sun?"

"Was not the cat the giver of all life?"

"Did not the cat hold man's destiny in his tiny paw?"

Cleopatra's Egypt no longer exists for the cat to purr about, but many of the animal behaviorists and pet owners I talked to feel that the modern feline still accepts the ancient theory that says, *"The cat is indeed sacred!"* Perhaps he is justified in believing in his omnipotence, for man has constantly tried to eliminate him, but has always failed.

The cat has rarely known a peaceful existence like

the dog's and has always had enemies. One of the severest enemies was Pope Gregory XI, who in the thirteenth century said that cats were used in pagan rites and were closely associated with the devil. He ordered his followers to "burn to death" the hated animal. In the fifteenth century, Pope Innocent VIII commanded believers to "rid the world of sorcerer cats," because they had some of the devil in them. Again the edict failed to have the desired effect and cats continued to multiply.

In the seventeenth century, according to Dr. Neil Todd, of the Carnivore Genetics Research Center in Newtonville, Massachusetts, cats were imported to the United States. Our country had a large rat population, and the cats proved to be very potent rat destroyers; they were chiefly used for that purpose for years. False legends sprang up which discouraged people from taking cats into their homes and trying to make pets out of them. *It couldn't be done!* was the claim. The chief old wives tales were:

• A cat will suck a baby's breath and strangle him.

• A cat is a solitary animal and dislikes humans intensely.

• Bad luck is sure to come to the individual who has a black cat cross his path.

Gradually, these myths were disproved and the cat became a pet. Today, there are 10 million cats in American homes and the prediction is that by the year 2000 that number will double. The reasons for the sudden ardor for cats are many, but the chief one I kept hearing is that they are "easy to love."

"Easy to love" becomes even easier when communication exists between owner and cat. And it can be done.

Cats, like human babies, come in all shapes and sizes: big, medium, small, skinny, fat, plain, pretty, simple, complex, mercurial, outgoing, contemplative. Regardless of appearance, breed, or intellect, most of them have one thing in common: the ability to communicate like very young children. Scientists have discovered that by applying the same method that has long been used successfully by adults to understand and communicate with their offspring, cat owners can be taught to carry on effective two-way conversations with their pets.

On a recent Tuesday morning Evelyn Miller of Cleveland, Ohio, scored a double victory. She succeeded in teaching both her ten-month-old daughter, Tish, and the family's seventh-month-old alley cat, Dibbie, to understand the word *catch*. As was her custom, the pleased woman rewarded her two pupils, but this time she made a slight mistake. She gave her daughter a cat biscuit and her cat a piece of zwieback. Apparently, the error didn't faze the recipients and, judging by their pleasure as they swiftly devoured the prizes, the linguistic lesson had been a great triumph.

Unfortunately, the joyful scene ended a few minutes later when Tish started crying and frantically heaving her shoulders. Mrs. Miller immediately knew that the child didn't have a bellyache because of the cat biscuit;

Tish was communicating her personal discomfort in a completely different area. She was saying, non-verbally, "My diaper is wet! Change it!" Her mother replied, verbally, "Hold everything, here I come!" She promptly replaced the diaper with a dry one and her daughter's crying and shoulder movement stopped.

Then the Ohio housewife started cleaning the house and turned on the vacuum cleaner. This time it was the cat's turn to howl. She started miaowing furiously and lifting her left paw up and down. The cat was saying, non-verbally, **"That darn noise is driving me nuts! I want out!"** Mrs. Miller turned off the vacuum cleaner and said, verbally, "Okay. Okay. You can play in the yard." She opened the back door and the miaowing and paw lifting ceased.

Barbara Austin, a director of the Dawn Animal Agency, which rescues hundreds of no longer wanted animals, is a leading authority on the care and treatment of cats and agrees heartily with Mrs. Miller's method. "Cat owners," Ms. Austin told me, "will be successful if they realize that the same set of standards that apply to children apply to cats. There are at least four 'freedom' rules that cat owners should adopt:

"1. Freedom for your cat to explore his own world.
"2. Freedom to develop at his own rate of speed.
"3. Freedom to make mistakes.
"4. Freedom to be loved even though those mistakes are committed."

The scientists I interviewed felt that owners should get to know a bit about the various breeds. Here are some of the main ones:

Silver tabby. This breed is the most common variety found in American homes, and is also often referred to as "alley cat." He is a mixed breed and short-haired. Frequently, he is striped and has a broad face, large expressive eyes, and is well-built. This breed varies greatly in characteristics and requires close, close observation on the part of the owner if two-way conversation is desired. Many silver tabby cats toss their tails straight up in the air when they want to say, "I'm very happy!"

Siamese. He is short-haired, medium-sized, slim, and comes in a variety of colors: tan, brown, blue, purple (yes, purple), red, and marked. His rear legs are a bit longer than the front ones. His eyes are wide set and slant slightly. One owner told me that this breed often looks like an Oriental Jackie Kennedy Onassis. He is said to be super-intelligent and the owner should have little trouble learning how to communicate with him, as he is prepared to discuss anything, including the state of the world. He can be very friendly and loves to hear words of praise regarding his charm or athletic ability.

Abyssinian. This breed looks like cats found on ancient Egyptian walls. He doesn't make friends easily, but when he is sure of your affection, you usually have a lifetime chum. A good way of getting that affection is by stroking and petting, *but let him make the decision when that should be!* He is a very fickle creature and petting at the wrong time can have an adverse effect. He is a very shy cat and you can help cure that shyness by trying never to leave him totally alone. That doesn't mean you need be at his side constantly, but you or some other person should always be within easy reach.

European short hair. Although he is referred to as a European breed many of his offspring are living in the United States. He is of medium height, sturdy, broad-chested, and has a long tail flared at the tip. He may pretend aloofness, but really desires company—and for some strange reason he seems to prefer women to men. A European short hair frequently hides the moment he hears the word "No." Therefore, one effective way to train him is to remove in advance any bric-a-brac that you are fearful he might break.

Manx. I was once offered a Manx kitten on the Isle of Man, which is supposed to be the origin of this once rare cat. The owner of the mother cat said to me, "They make good, sensible pets if you don't expect too much." His advice was sound because others have said much the same. "Live and let live," seems to be this cat's motto. This breed doesn't have a tail and makes up for it by expressing himself by exaggerated body movements. A lifting of the front paws usually means, **"Let's play"** and swinging on the back paws often can be interpreted as, **"Think of a new game to play!"**

Persian. Shirley MacLaine, the Hollywood actress, said that she wore her hair short because when it was long it required as much grooming as a Persian cat. And that's a lot! This cat has long, silky hair that needs constant combing. The result is very lovely to look at and some owners are content with the cat's splendid appearance. So the cat tends to grow lazy and increase its food intake—and the new fat cat becomes even lazier. The "good" owner doesn't allow this to happen and talks and plays with his cat often. Persians communicate frequently through movements of the eyes, which are blue or green. They are a very provocative breed and require firm but gentle treatment. Repetition is quite necessary—start with easy words like *food* and *ball.*

For some strange reason people insist on giving foreign breeds outlandish names. When they do, the cat will usually raise an objection; it may be subtle, but it's ever present. Animal authority Cleveland Amory tells of a case where two cats rebelled by not responding.

"Many men and women give their cats names that are too hard—or not hard enough," he said. "What you need are distinctive-sounding names. Cats in general are very sensitive to sound and will surely understand whatever name you give them, even if they also want you to understand that they don't want to answer to it."

One owner told Amory that she named her two kittens Topaz and Amber because of the color of their eyes. The kittens didn't like the names and refused to reply when called them. The woman then tried Martini and Manhattan. Again they refused.

"In desperation," says Amory, "she tried calling one

kitten O'Shaughnessy. It worked. But the other kitten was stubborn. No matter what name the woman tried, nothing seemed to suit the cat. While the struggle was going on, the kitten acted so funny that one day the woman happened to say, 'You're *silly.*' Immediately, that name stuck."

The conclusion that Amory drew from this and from similar incidents is that a cat will accept or reject the name you give, depending on whether or not he likes the sound of it. He's a very independent creature—and that's his charm. Be prepared to live with it—not change it!

Can cats be trained? Or do you have to accept a cat strictly on its own terms—human hands completely off? Dr. Leon F. Whitney, a Connecticut veterinarian who has treated thousands of cats, says, "Almost everyone mistakenly believes that cats are elegant parasites that can't be trained. They can, and almost as easily as dogs. However, cats cannot be trained by force, but only with the patient application of refined principles (as befits a cat's image) of modern psychology. By tempting a cat to behave in a certain way and then rewarding it for doing so, you can 'condition' its activities."

Dr. Whitney, who directs the largest pet clinic in the East, adds, "The key to effective conditioning is teaching a cat to associate a sound with satisfaction."

Recently, whether they're aware of it or not, cats received a tremendous boost in status when one of their number became a famous TV personality. Until then, Lassie, the collie, refused to share the center of the stage with any feline. Now, Morris, the superstar of the pet food commercial, is in great demand—he's even "authorized" a biography in which he discusses his love life and delivers candid opinions on the human world.

Like all make-believe, the qualities attributed to Lassie and Morris by their managers contain some elements of truth. Animal behaviorists have discovered that your cat, indeed, does have definite thoughts and is eager to share them with you. Let's meet some owners who have learned how to converse with their cats.

CHAPTER VII

Successful
Cat Owners Explain
How They Communicate
with Their Pets

Montaigne, the sixteenth-century French essayist and acute observer of felines, once wrote, "Cats undoubtedly talk and reason among themselves." For hundreds of years the statement was accepted as definitive, but recently authorities have added the phrase, "... *and with people!*"

This important supplement originated with observers who explain that by carefully watching a cat's ever-changing expression and by listening to its miaowing and purring they have learned how to interpret what it is saying. Many scientists and cat authorities confirm this.

Gillette Grilhé, a graduate of the Sorbonne and an outstanding authority, has written extensively about man's relationship with cats. Her current book, *The Cat and Man,* is regarded as a classic in the cat world. She says, "There is no doubt that he [the cat] has a language for communicating with man. . . ."

The men and women in the following reports—all cat owners—told me emphatically that they are accustomed to conversing with their pets all the time. In each case, town officials and neighbors vouched for the integrity and veracity of these cat lovers, although I think it only fair to tell you that I have found most cat owners—this group included—to be in a class by themselves. They make all other pet owners sound positively bored when it comes to discussing animal intelligence. They aren't kidding when they say their very particular cat is "truly God's gift to man."

They mean every word of it. I had never been the world's greatest cat booster but I confess that time and time again I was amazed as I watched them carry on two-way conversations with their pets. I urged some of these people to tell you about the psychology behind communication and cats, and they were delighted to have the opportunity to expound on this subject.

Mrs. Blassingame and the Tape Recorder

Ever since childhood, Selma Blassingame had suffered from a severe case of asthma. She was diagnosed as being "allergic to cats." Keep far away from them, the doctors had instructed her. Mrs. Blassingame wasn't happy about this medical recommendation. She had always been extremely fond of cats. "Puss and Boots was my all-time favorite story," she told me.

Luckily, shortly after her marriage to a former oil

driller who had struck it rich and now owns three supermarkets, her wheezing and all other signs of asthma vanished—and she celebrated by getting a rare and lovely Abyssinian cat. The asthma didn't return.

The Blassingames and their two children live in a many-gabled Victorian house near Toledo, Ohio. "Other than my owning three cats," she said, "I am quite ordinary. I go to church on Sunday; I watch 'Marcus Welby, M.D.,' on Tuesday; I play bridge on Thursday; and I bake bread on Friday—sometimes I get real daring and bake whole-wheat loaves instead of white. Some daring! My husband says I've developed into a real stick-in-the-mud."

But with her cats, Mrs. Blassingame is far from dull. I watched her get down on hands and knees as she invented unconventional games to play with her three pets. They seemed to prefer close contact contests. One popular game involved Mrs. Blassingame balancing a cat on her back and bucking violently. The cat who held on the longest was declared the winner. They enjoyed this game tremendously and "laughed" as they demanded more. (Yes, I did say laugh. Not the way you and I do, but the cats definitely made chuckling sounds, and I never drink alcohol during work.)

The sounds varied with each cat and several times Mrs. Blassingame stressed that fact. "They have distinct personalities," she said. The cats, too, seemed to be aware of it. They were all present in the living room while I was conducting the interview and all were doing different things: one snored contentedly as he dozed on my lap, one paced back and forth while muttering to himself, and one stared at the twenty-four-inch television screen although the set wasn't turned on.

Successful Cat Owners Communicate with Their Pets

They only performed alike when the children came home from school. Joan, aged fourteen, put out a gigantic bowl of milk and all the cats immediately rushed toward it. I watched as they drank greedily, and, when they felt they had enough, they lay down on the wall-to-wall living room carpet, tucked their paws in, and curled their tails around their bodies. It was evident that they were contented.

Selma Blassingame: "I tried to make myself understood to Viva, the first cat I owned after my asthma had disappeared, but, somehow, I didn't have any luck. Although I seemed to comprehend a little of what she was saying, nothing that I did could get her to understand me. It got to the point where I thought she was just plain stupid—and that I was stupid for wanting to own a cat!

"That was when my sister Maria said, 'Selma, you always jabber to her in an excited tone. You ought to hear yourself—that is if you could even make out yourself what you're saying.'

"My husband uses a tape recorder occasionally for his correspondence and I borrowed it. Maria was right! I sounded like Minnie Mouse with a bad bellyache! No wonder Viva didn't understand me. She'd have to be a genius to know what I was saying. From that day on I deliberately began speaking clearly, distinctly and in an easy, calm voice. That seemed to change things drastically and Viva suddenly knew what I was saying.

"She died two years ago. Although we live on a side street and have a full-stop sign on the corner, cars come zooming along and one of those speed demons ran over

Viva. We rushed her to the veterinarian, but he said it would be impossible for her to ever again live a normal life. The accident had caused a complete paralysis of her nervous system. We put her to rest and were grateful that it didn't hurt her. Fortunately, it is now possible to give the cat a painless injection that stops life instantly.

"Since Viva's tragic accident I've seen to it that the other cats never wander onto the road. I keep them in our backyard. We put screening on top of the fence and we constantly check for holes.

"I had been so pleased with Viva's progress in communicating that I started acquiring other cats and conversing with them. At present I have two Persians and a long-haired chinchilla. I'm constantly learning from them.

"They have taught me the value of privacy. I was always a gregarious person and felt that I always had to be around people. My cats have shown me how solitude can have a really soothing effect. Perhaps one of the reasons for my asthma was that I felt that I was personally accountable for the moods of others. If my parents or sister were down in the dumps I thought it was because of me and that it was my responsibility to cheer them up. My cats have shown me otherwise. Oh, they cheer me up all right. But they don't act as if it's their sole function.

"I discovered years ago that just a little thing like a tape recorder can work cat miracles. Probably because they hear things again and again, cats will suddenly latch on to the idea of what you're saying. You don't need a large parcel of tricks to train a cat to converse with you. They confide many things: who they like, what they like, and how they like it.

"Cats are not the strange and mysterious creatures that legend would have you believe. I know a cat can exist without human care, but I'm sure the cat wouldn't like it at all. No matter what you hear to the contrary, believe this—cats like humans who like them!

"One of the most frequent myths I've heard is that cats are not trainable. I say, '*Hogwash!*' to that theory. I suppose if you want a really well-trained cat you've got to start when he's still a very tiny kitten. But it's really never too late to stop him from clawing on furniture or keep him from roaming too far—things like that. If you're willing to take the time on his training I can almost promise extravagant results. I've even heard of many cases where the cat has been trained to a leash, to heel and sit. *That myth about cats being untrainable is spread by dog owners!*"

"*In Vietnam I Learned to Use Body Language*"

Gail Moreso lives in a New York brownstone house that has been nominated for landmark status. It was lavishly built at the turn of the century and was recently restored to its former elegance. Gail likes living in the house and evidently so does her year-old Siamese cat. "Cats have definite architectural tastes," she said. "I used to live in Greenwich Village and the cat I owned at the time didn't approve of the apartment. I swear he would stick his tongue out and issue a loud Bronx cheer!"

Gail was born in New Rochelle, but has lived in New

York City since 1955, when she started attending nurses' training school. She graduated in 1959 and worked in a hospital for nine years. In 1968 she decided that her nursing talents would be helpful in Vietnam and volunteered her services. She knew that the Vietnamese people desperately needed help, but discovered that often the help worked in reverse.

"I think that many Americans who go to places like Vietnam," said the pretty, slender nurse, "often find it difficult to accept the country's standards and values. They seem to be sorry that they can't give the best of our care and culture."

Gail quickly learned that many other people have something valuable to offer us. "Often it might be something simple but still important—like their high regard for pets. They really do talk to them."

It was in Vietnam that Gail was made aware of how much of language is non-verbal. "I'd carry on involved conversations without knowing any of the spoken language. But a grimace, a pointed finger, a sudden shake of the shoulders, I discovered, are also an important part of communication." When Gail returned to the United States she used that knowledge on her cats and again it worked. She understood them—and what's more she could now make her speech comprehensible to them.

Gail Moreso: "Cats have an ability to let you think that you are extra-special. Granted, this may not be constant, but it happens often enough to make me feel very glad that I own one. My cat is passionate, uninhibited, beautiful, affectionate . . . I could go on and on.

"People have a lot of strange notions about cats. One

is that they just can't remember. That isn't so and I can tell from first-hand experience. When I went to Vietnam I gave my Siamese away. When I returned I visited the friend I had given the cat to, and I was astounded by the royal greeting the cat gave me. He purred and purred and kept swishing his tail frantically. He kept following me around and didn't want me to go to the bathroom. I knew he was saying, '**How wonderful it is to see you again! Where have you been?**'

"When I get a new cat, one of the initial things I do is to bend down to his level. Cats seem to realize that you're doing something out of the ordinary, so they respond appreciatively. I have found that they acknowledge your desire to meet them at least halfway by trying to cooperate.

"Then I tell him how glad I am that he's there. I repeat the words over and over, but often that isn't enough—my eyes, face, hands also join the conversation. Soon, he understands what I am saying, a gentle purring is the tip-off.

"Another thing I do may be called *doing nothing.* Cats are very sensitive and don't react well to punishment. As a matter of fact, punishment often limits or ends communication. Long ago, I learned that where cats are concerned it's difficult to keep certain things off-limits. Sure, I had some items broken, but you'd be surprised how few. A cat is very careful and won't deliberately want to break things. But when he does, he will try to deny it, especially if it happens while you're away.

"He more than makes up for it when you return. When I get home and find myself tired after a trying day that's when I find his greeting most worthwhile. I have gone back to school and, as you know, some professors really load the work on. The cat senses when I need cheering up and acts accordingly. Sometimes I come home in such a foul mood that I take it out on him. Instead of saying, 'How nice to see you,' in a tone that really means it, I growl. Before I have a chance to finish, he senses it and runs under the couch. But after a few seconds he comes out and confronts me. I feel so ashamed that I begin to play with him.

"He loves TV and his favorite program is watching the Knicks play basketball. I believe it's the fast action that intrigues him. He'll climb up on top of the set, lie down on his back, and view it in an inverted position.

"You get so attuned to an animal that you're almost on his wave-length. You may think that's strange, but about a week before my last cat died—he wasn't ill—I left him in care of a trusted friend and went away for the weekend. The first day I was there I sensed that the cat was in trouble; the feeling became stronger and stronger. 'Am I fantasizing and becoming a worrisome crank?' I kept asking myself. I don't usually have these strange premonitions. It was actually the first time I've had such feelings.

"During the night those thoughts became almost unbearable. I was glad when morning finally arrived. I couldn't get home fast enough. My cat was fine, but I was so glad to see him that I gave him an extra-special meal and played with him for a long time. Over the next few days we were very close and I guess I was more affectionate than usual.

"I relish the thought that I had the opportunity, because just a week after that strange premonition the

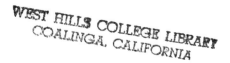

cat died. I'm certain that cats use ESP for communication."

The Cat Who Helped Make
Retirement Worthwhile

When Martin Anderson retired from his civil service job in Washington, D.C., he and his wife, Betty, envisioned a leisurely future of traveling, gardening, and bowling. During the first two months they visited their married daughter in Houston, and on the way back stopped at the Grand Canyon; planted dozens of bulbs and herbs in their backyard garden; went bowling twice a week.

"What with my pension and savings," Martin told me, "everything looked rosy, but after twenty-four years of an eight-to-four routine I felt really guilty about 'doing nothing.' What's more, I was plain bored!" That's when Martin Anderson took a part-time job as a cashier in a local shoe store and adopted a three-week-old kitten.

"You wouldn't believe the change it made," Betty Anderson said. "Martin is sixty-nine years old, but suddenly he looked and acted like a man ten years younger." Then she winked as she added, "I suppose that running after the cat is what keeps him fit."

The Andersons live on the south side of the nation's capital. They were going to sell their house and rent an apartment, but, after hearing about current prices, they decided to turn their sixty-five-year-old house into a two-family dwelling. They figured that with Martin doing all the alterations the rent would pay for the taxes and upkeep.

Martin had polio when he was a child and it affected his right leg—he still drags it slightly. But other than that mild deformity his doctor has declared him in perfect shape, although he said he smokes too much. I watched Martin do some carpentering on the new apartment—he was puffing a fat cigar. Rudder, the cat, also watched and every once in a while she would miaow loudly as if she were making a suggestion. Martin seemed to respond to her criticism. Once he muttered out loud, "Okay, I'll put that damn beam over there. Satisfied?" Since the cat and I were the only ones present and since I hadn't said anything . . .

Martin Anderson: "There were two things that I really believe helped tremendously in making me able to talk to my cat: keeping a notebook and using a mirror. That may sound like a lot of crap, but that's just what I did—and what's more, that 'crap' worked.

"Well, to start with, I never had a cat until I got Rudder. I had dogs when I was a kid—there was a Boston bull that I remember and also a mongrel named Lefty. Why he was called Lefty I never could figure out; it seemed to me that he favored his right side. Well, you can't account for some things and I suppose that's good.

"They weren't really my dogs—they belonged to the whole family. And I can't honestly say that I ever talked to them or that they understood me. It was a case of their always being around and I didn't ever question it. After them, a hell of a long time went by without my having any kind of a pet. That was when Rudder came along.

"I'm rushing the story. For years, I was a clerk in the Government Printing Office and I decided the time had come to retire. I had been thinking about it for quite a while; guys in the office who were younger than me were retiring left and right. Hell, I could have continued working at least three more years. At first, things went along fine, but then Betty started complaining that I was getting restless. I found a job as a relief cashier in a shoe store. I'd work two nights a week and also when the regular cashier was away on vacation. That helped, but I still didn't solve the whole problem.

"Our neighbors had a cat and their cat had kittens. The next thing I knew, Betty and I decided to take one of the kittens. The only thing I knew about cats was something I once read in a book—that male cats were supposed to roam more and were more independent. So we chose a she-kitten. Only that's not so easy to know when they're young. I found out how it's done—you pick up the tail and if you see kind of a dot then it's a he, but if the dot has a horizontal line below it, then it's a she. If you have real doubts, I suggest you consult a veterinarian.

"Did you ever see a very young kitten up close? This one was three weeks old and Betty said that it looked like the sweetest and most innocent thing that ever lived. The kitten already had been given the name Rudder and I suppose we found it easy to keep it. The neighbor who owned the cat litter is a real boat nut; he keeps a twenty-five-footer in his driveway. He named the others with nautical terms also: Starboard, Port, Head. Me, I prefer to leave boats strictly alone—I get seasick just from taking a paddleboat on the Potomac!

"We took Rudder to the vet a couple of weeks later

and he gave her some shots. She's been a healthy cat and the only other time we had to take her to the vet was when she was spayed. Betty and I had a real brouhaha over that one. She was for spaying. Me, I said that it was only natural for Rudder to have a normal sex life; why shouldn't the cat enjoy herself? After arguing for days we came to a compromise: Rudder would have one litter and then be spayed.

"She had her kittens a couple of years ago—blooming and vigorous kittens, but even then we had trouble finding potential owners. For one of them we couldn't find a home no matter how hard we tried. We were going to have him put to sleep, but we didn't have the heart for it and fortunately my sister and brother-in-law took him. See, even brother-in-laws are good for something. Incidentally, he gave me some good advice about the cat. He told me that if I wanted to avoid having my sofa and other good furniture scratched raw, I should provide a scratching post—a simple round bowl enclosed by a piece of carpet remnant. I showed Rudder how to use the post, and ever since she's kept pretty clear of our furniture.

"Now, I finally come to the part about communication. Like I said, there were two things that stand out and they're really simple, too.

"I have a terrible memory. Betty says that if my shirt wasn't on my back, I'd forget where it was. When I was working for the government, my boss would always be rude to me about forgetting to put things in my reports. But he was the kind of a guy who would never get off his ass so I never paid him any attention. Anyway, I know I have a bad memory. As I get older it seems to be worse.

That's why I decided to keep a notebook full of Rudder's actions.

"When she jumped up on the kitchen counter and put out her paw, that always meant that she wanted to be fed. If she moved her tail up and down real hard and swayed her body from side to side it meant, '**The room's cold, turn the heat up.**' When she made herself stiff and her body started to shake it meant that she wanted me to play some soft music on the phonograph. Before I'd accept that one of Rudder's signals meant some definite thing, there would have to be at least five similar entries. Pretty soon I gathered a lot of them—you'd be surprised how many tell-tale signals a cat gives off. The trick is to remember them, so I found the notebook very worthwhile—at least for me.

"Then there's the mirror; that's even simpler than keeping a record. I found that out by sheer accident. We have one on our bedroom closet door and once when Rudder was in the room I made some funny faces in the mirror. Oh, things like putting my thumb in the corner of my mouth and stretching it. Popping my eyes out. Fingers on my nose.

"Rudder was standing behind me and saw my faces in the mirror. It was pretty obvious that she was enjoying my performance. I made the faces again and again. She looked amused. I didn't know why—maybe it was just plain curiosity—but I took Rudder away from the mirror and made those same faces; this time there was no response. I went back to the bedroom mirror and made the faces—again Rudder seemed real amused.

"That got me to thinking—evidently, she liked looking in the mirror. Why not use it to get words and sentences across? I started talking to her through the mirror and soon it worked like a charm.

"I'd look in the mirror and, for example, make signs signifying eating. I'd chomp my lips up and down and pretty soon Rudder was doing the same thing. Then I'd say the word 'Eat' over and over. Or I'd say, 'Close eyes,' and shut and open my eyes. Rudder loves to imitate everything I do and she would do the same thing.

"But I didn't always make signs. Often I'd just point to something and repeat it about a dozen times. 'Trousers,' 'pillow,' 'bed,' 'window,' 'door.' . . . You just name it and it's now in Rudder's vocabulary. She really caught on. I found out that the trick is that when you make use of the mirror you have to be sure that you're pointing exactly to the item you want her to learn and then to keep reiterating it in a very loud and clear voice.

"Don't ask me why it worked. I don't have any formal answers, but don't they say that cats are mysterious? The mirror has another important function—it helps me to see the way I look to her."

CHAPTER VIII

More
Cat Owners Explain

The Cats Who Like Franz Schubert

Joy and Patrick McGinnis plus their six cats make a very musical family. Patrick is the former manager of New York's Avery Fisher Hall and is a gifted pianist. His wife, Joy, has a fine mezzo-soprano voice and often the two give home recitals. Max, Cato, Lyle, Sussie, Ginnie, and Gladys—the six cats—listen to the couple's music and are a very appreciate audience, but occasionally they protest and miaow loudly when the compositions of Franz Schubert are not included.

Music is one of the bonds that drew the McGinnises together, and the love of cats helped cement the relationship.

"I'm sure that I would have given my cats away if Packy hadn't liked them," Joy said. "But it would have been with great reluctance—and it sure helped when I learned that he felt as strongly about them as I did."

Joy feels that she has always been able to communicate with her cats, but that the comprehension really increased the more she applied herself. "I suppose it's like knowing a musical score. You think you know all about it, then you start practicing and discover that there's a great deal you have yet to learn. You play it over and over and then, wham, you suddenly have it. Well, it's the same way with cats—practice makes perfect!"

When you talk to Joy McGinnis it soon becomes obvious that she is a professional singer; her speaking voice is very melodious and has a resonant ring to it. She enunciates each word clearly and carefully. She has found that the cats respond best when she does that. She could not be described as a rare beauty, but after being in her presence for just a brief time you are aware that the tall, slender, middle-aged woman has a captivating aura about her, and the cats seem to sense that, too.

She spoke to me about cats in her large New York City apartment. The living room is lined with books devoted to music and also contains Packy's huge grand piano. The cats know that the furnishings are to be avoided, but everything else is part of their domain.

Joy McGinnis: "After you phoned me I started to pay special attention to cat communication. Before that I guess I just took it for granted. It seems to me that some phase of communication starts early in the morning when Packy and I get up and some of it goes on until we're ready to turn in. I don't mean to imply that the cats are constantly under foot—they sleep a great deal—but when they're around one of them always seems to be saying something. Unlike other animals, cats don't select a single spokesman—they're all individualists and *all* of them have something to say.

"During the week we use an alarm clock–radio to get us out of bed. And the moment the cats hear the announcer's voice—he may be selling used cars—they feel it's a signal for me to fetch their breakfast. If we happen to sleep late on a Saturday or Sunday, they stand at the foot of the bed and stare. You may be sound asleep, but not for long when twelve eyes are riveted to your face. Their eyes are very expressive and the message is clear: **'It's time to rise and shine!'**

"From that moment on, the eyes and the rest of their bodies start speaking. Perhaps Cato looks very guilty as his eyes widen and his fur stands up slightly. That's a sign that he's been up to some mischief. I ask him what he's done, and his eyes grow wider and the fur stands further up. This is how he tells me that during the night he probably clawed on one of the chairs. I look at them and, sure enough, one bears fresh scratches.

"Cato promptly scoots off, although he knows that I won't dole out punishment. Long ago I learned that there's no point in using punishment unless the culprit is actually caught in the act. When I see them do something I object to, I chase after them, but under no circumstances do I ever hit them. All that punishment seems to accomplish is to make both cat and owner unhappy, and *the cat is rarely cured of performing the unwanted act.* If you do *succeed* by using *cruel* punishment, the cat will not forget what you've done, and you may have made an enemy for life. Cats, like elephants, have long memories.

"Most cats are frightened by sudden noise and when

that happens I invariably lift the cat up and pet him. When I put him down he always rubs against my leg, and I know that he's saying: **'Thanks for caring.'**

"They will often tell you about their likes and dislikes. Lyle prefers a certain brand of food and when he desperately wants it he goes to the garbage can and empties the contents on the floor. His message is quite clear: **'I want what I want.'**

"If Packy and I stay up late, Cato starts pacing from room to room. We know he, too, is telling us something: **'Go to bed so that I can turn in also—I've had a hard day! Be reasonable!'** He never goes to sleep until we do and, when we finally turn out all the lights, he purrs contentedly. Again we know what he's saying: **'Thanks, but it's about time. I'll turn in now.'**

"When I go to the closet and pull down a carrier case, suddenly all six cats disappear because they know that one of them is going to the vet—and no one wants to be that one. *As I said, cats are very, very clever animals!*"

The Professor's Advice

Philosopher Bertrand Russell once said, "An attractive teacher makes learning attractive." Lord Russell must have been envisioning someone like Sara Barnhart because she fits his description completely. Dr. Barnhart is a young, gorgeous, blonde communications teacher at New York's Queens College. Her classes usually enjoy 100 percent attendance because the students always find her lectures informative and they get a special bonus of having them delivered by a lovely-looking woman.

Although Dr. Barnhart is only in her late twenties, she is considered an authority on many phases of communication. Knowing that, I decided to interview her, and when I asked her whether humans can converse with cats, she replied promptly and emphatically: "Absolutely!"

What makes her comments even more meaningful is that Dr. Barnhart is also a cat owner. She acquired two-year-old Pooh when he was a tiny kitten, and has been delighted with his presence ever since. "I talk to Pooh constantly," Dr. Barnhart said. "That's only natural—he's my friend, and you talk to friends."

Sara Barnhart: "In human communication, I tell you verbally that I want to do something and explain what it is. For instance: suppose you understand what I mean, but you say: 'For the following reasons I can't do it right now.' There we have one of the major communication differences between humans and animals. The cat can't tell you why he won't do something. Oh, there are exceptions to that rule—for example, the cat refuses to go outside because it's raining. He looks at the falling drops and then at you, and he is conveying: **'Only a fool would go out in weather like this.'** *And he certainly isn't a fool!*

"I can attest to that. Pooh knows my ritual in the morning and doesn't do anything until he hears me turn off the hair dryer—that's the signal for his asking for cereal. He does this by coming into the bathroom, rubbing against my leg, and miaowing. He seldom makes noise, so I'm instantly alert to his demand. As a matter of fact, the only other time he miaows is when he sees bugs—that really sets him off. But even then the miaowing is firm but gentle; he relies heavily on body language. Humans depend on it, too. You'd be surprised at the large amount of non-verbal 'speaking' we do. A large amount of information regarding the emotional state of a human speaker is conveyed not so much by his words, but by his actions. I often tell my students to note the number of times a day they use body language. That's a good exercise to use; try it for fifteen minutes or a half-hour. Don't use your voice, just your body. I'll wager you can make yourself understood.

"Animals probably communicate fear, anger, sadness, and joy in the same way that we do. I don't mean that a very sad cat will start to cry and beat his chest, but it becomes very apparent when the cat is dejected. His face often contains the same expressions that human faces possess during such moments. The same thing applies to the other three emotions.

"I've discovered that when Pooh is joyful his eyes open wide and his face radiates glee and pleasure. When he is mad or worried he really frowns. A friend of mine who helped us celebrate his birthday said, 'I don't think Pooh likes getting older—he looks so worried.' *Yes, the cat was frowning.*

"There are two things that Pooh can't do in the house. They are: interfering with my sleep and playing with the house plants. The way I cured him of committing those two offenses was by using a spritzer, a kind of water pistol. Every time he got me out of bed or played with the plants I let him have it between the eyes; he stopped doing them very soon.

"Other times I don't punish him although I have been somewhat annoyed by his treatment of the toilet paper; he pulls the roll out into long strips. I'll be working at my desk and I hear him playing with the toilet paper. I'll shout 'No! Stop it!' But that doesn't work. After a while I get up and remove him physically. But he often goes back. I suppose the reason is simple—he knows it makes me angry and I must have done something earlier to annoy him.

"He is a quick study and there are many things he learns in a hurry. Pooh loves to go out, and, since I live in a garden apartment, he can get out frequently. I noticed that he would respond to my suggestion when he was only several months old. 'Pooh,' I'd say, 'do you want to go outside?' Perhaps it was because of body language on my part that he understood so early. I'd ask it verbally, but unconsciously I'd move toward the door, and that may have tipped him off. He could have noticed that slight move and associated it with the verbal message.

"Another thing Pooh learned quickly was to associate a suitcase with departure. When he'd see me packing he instantly knew I was going away and that would mean someone else would be taking care of him. He'd show his displeasure by running into the bathroom and playing with the toilet paper. Even a change of dress makes him aware that something's about to happen. I'll come home from school and put on a different skirt and blouse, and Pooh instantly knows that I'm going out and will be away several hours.

"Soft or harsh verbal tones indicate how humans feel, and cats do exactly the same thing. For some reason, Pooh prefers my female friends—it may be that they're nicer to him and that he knows them better. Whatever the reason, he greets them effusively and nuzzles close to them or sits in their laps. The only time one of my female friends confused him somewhat is when she read *Winnie the Pooh* to her young daughter in his presence. Every time she came to the word 'Pooh' my Pooh would respond instantly, but my friend would ignore him. Finally, in desperation, the cat knocked the book out of her hands.

"She learned the hard way that you can't ignore a cat!"

"If My Trixie Likes You, Then You Must Be Okay"

Lenore Faubel, who lives in Lincoln, Nebraska, has a simple rule that she applies to people: if her cat likes you, then she does too. If Trixie doesn't, then there's obviously something radically wrong with you.

Mrs. Faubel is a masseuse. She works at home, and a large part of the first floor is sectioned off by metal bars for her work room. Trixie, a six-year-old white Angora cat, is urged to stay away, but occasionally her outgoing disposition causes her to climb up on one of the poles and peer inside. About a fourth of her face—including a small part of one eye—is barely visible. Long-time clients are not too surprised when they see the white sliver. They've learned that it's Trixie's way of saying, **"Hello, I'm glad to see you."**

Clarence Faubel, Lenore's late husband, was a concert violinist and died many years ago. Since then, his widow has resided in Lincoln with a cat by her side. "It seems that all my life," she said, "I've had a cat around, and each one appears to be more intelligent than the last—we talk more extensively. Perhaps it has something to do with age; humans, like good wine, are supposed to improve with time."

Lenore Faubel: "I grew up on a farm about 150 miles west of here and the nearest child who was my age was quite distant. But that didn't stop me from telling my mother that I was going outdoors. Then I'd wheel my doll carriage outside.

"I'd quickly run to the barn to fetch my cat, Belle, put her in the doll carriage, and wheel her around. Belle and I'd have such fun. I was careful to do it on the north side of the house, which was out of my mother's view, because she didn't like cats nohow.

"Mother didn't mince words. 'I'll tolerate these critters only in the barn,' she'd say to my father. 'Those sneaky varmints are only good for mouse catching. I don't want them running through my house!'

"During one cold winter I saw a strange cat bogged down in the snow. I couldn't take him to the barn because the snow was over my head, so I softly sneaked the cat inside the house and put him in the cellar. I put my finger to my lips and said, 'Sh-sh-sh.' He didn't understand what I meant, and he miaowed. Quickly, I placed my hand over his mouth and once again I said, 'Sh-sh-sh.' Thank goodness he figured out what I was saying.

"I guess that was when I became aware that cats can understand people—*if the people just try to be understood!* Ever since that day I have had meaningful conversations with my cats.

"After all, they're like children, and I suppose that's the secret behind getting them to communicate. Apply the same rules in bringing up cats that you'd use with children. Trixie gets her food on time, she's taken care of when she's sick; she knows what she can do and can't; and she gets plenty of love.

"Maybe the last one is the most important. My husband used to raise St. Bernards and I know that he was extremely fond of them, but I don't think I can remember a single time when Clarence told them so. I've discovered that with animals, especially with cats, you've got to tell them and show them how you feel. Once or twice isn't enough—you got to do it often!

"It pays off and you get lots of dividends that way. When I'm feeling blue, Trixie comforts me. When I come home she greets me. When I go to sleep she bids me goodnight. I have to admit that it took some effort to get her to do those things, but it was worth it. She always seemed to sense when I was feeling blue. She'd jump into my lap at those times but she'd quickly jump out. I wanted her consolation and would clutch her tightly. Evidently that didn't please her—she wanted to be the giver. So I learned to sit still and allow her to make the advances. With cats that's very important to understand: *they don't want a boss—just a friend.*

"When I'd come home after a day in town, I learned to get down and pet her and at the same time say in a gentle tone, 'How very nice to be with you. You're a wonderful cat!' Then, quickly, I'd get a goodie.

"The goodnight routine was a little harder. I had to work on that for a long time and, try as I would, nothing seemed to be happening. She just wouldn't say anything when I went to sleep. Then, by sheer accident one night, I yawned and said, 'I'm sorry, but I must be real sleepy. I'm going off to bed.' That yawn did it. Suddenly Trixie looked as if she comprehended what I'd been asking her to do. Her ears went back and she bobbed her head curtly up and down. Her motions seemed to signify the final acts of the day. So I learned that you can't rush a cat. They'll do what you want, but in their own sweet time.

"I've trained Trixie to tell me when someone is at the door. The way I did that was to ring the bell and then race upstairs. I did this over and over and pretty soon Trixie got it. Now, when I'm upstairs and don't hear the bell—I may be sitting at the dressing table—Trixie will race upstairs and come right over to me. She begins to miaow, then looks up and begins to frown. Her pupils grow larger and her ears wiggle back and forth. I know she is saying, '**Why don't you answer the door?**'

"I don't want you to think that it was always perfectly serene. Far from it. Although I'd had a lot of cats before Trixie, she sure got me down at the beginning. She'd run through the house as if wild horses were chasing her; she'd knock things about helter-skelter; she'd claw on furniture. I shouted 'No!' and hit her with a rolled-up newspaper, but it didn't help; *nothing did!* What in the world was I going to do?

"I think of myself as a religious person, and in desperation I turned to God and asked Him what to do. The answer came back rapidly: *Just love her a little more and let her know it.* So I switched courses. I didn't use the paper anymore. I didn't keep shouting 'No!' I used a kinder voice when I was talking to her. I lifted her up and petted her more often. And do you know what? *It worked! You can see for yourself how well it did!*"

"I Never Liked Cats Until . . ."

Katherine Coke is surrounded by extremely intelligent people, but still she stands out. Ms. Coke has climbed all the way up the success ladder and is now considered one of the smartest and most sagacious people in the media time-and-space-buying field. She spends more than $1 million a year purchasing radio advertising for the country's largest home-products organization.

One of her colleagues told me, "Kate is a super-bright person, and if she has taken a liking to cats then there has to be something special about them! Nobody, not even a cat, can fool Kate for very long!"

The interview was conducted in Ms. Coke's New York apartment. Both she and her home are very attractive.

Katherine Coke: "My son gave Lucifer to me as a Christmas present. 'Mom,' he said, 'I know how you feel about cats, but please give this little guy a chance before you make some negative comment. Please.'

"Reluctantly, I agreed. My son was constantly raving about his cat and felt that there was no greater cheerer-upper. I had always liked dogs and horses, definitely not cats—as far as I was concerned they were selfish, solitary, and sneaky. That sneaky part even affected the cat's sex. When Lucifer went to the veterinarian for initial shots, the vet said, 'I hate to tell you this, but your male is a female!' Talk about being shifty. I was a little shocked, but I decided to keep the cat and the name despite the sudden change of sex. At times Lucifer looks so evil—the epitome of the black cat. I simply added a middle name, Belle.

"Lucifer Belle is a pure Persian and is two years old. I suppose my first step in becoming a cat lover occurred a few minutes after she arrived. You can't resist a seven-week-old kitten very long—she was without doubt the prettiest thing I have ever seen. I found myself telling her that, and I believe she accepted me on those terms. Today, when I say, 'Lucifer Belle, are you a pretty kitty?' she'll immediately respond by wagging her tail to the right. She is saying, '**Yes, of course!**'

"I get the same response when I ask her, 'Do I love you?,' or 'Do you love me?' But there's no tail-wagging when I say, 'I'm not sure how I feel about you.' When she hears that she'll frown, raise her back, and disappear. But most of the time we get on just fine because I discovered the four *musts* for being a successful cat owner:

"1. Give the cat plenty of love.
"2. Talk to her—not gibberish, but real, honest-to-God conversation.
"3. Hold her—make her aware of your smell and feel.
"4. Play with her.

"Lucifer Belle's play period usually begins when I return from the office and lasts for about thirty minutes. One evening when I came home really tired I said,

'Lucifer Belle, I just haven't sufficient energy to play with you tonight.'

"She promptly lowered her ears and stiffened her tail—that's a sure sign that she's very sad. So we played and a few minutes later she kissed my cheek. Suddenly, all my tiredness disappeared.

"She's a great ham and loves to have her picture taken. As soon as a close friend of mine arrives Lucifer Belle starts posturing like some model for *Vogue,* hoping that he will snap her picture. I may not have liked cats once, but I sure do now, and I've found that the greater your rapport with them, the greater the love—both for owner and cat!"

CHAPTER IX

Communicating with Your Pet Bird

A recent poll reported that one out of every five families in the United States has at least one pet bird and that most of the owners are thoroughly delighted with their tiny winged friends' performances. Bird owners may not be quite as vociferous as cat owners, but they also make considerable claims for their pets. While writing this book I found that many of the boasts were quite accurate. Here are some remarkable feats that I observed or listened to:

• In Miami, Florida, a parakeet possessed a vocabulary of more than four hundred English and Yiddish phrases—and knew what many of them meant. Scoffers told me that a "talking" bird couldn't possibly reason, but merely mimicked and repeated words. Yet with this bird a specific word or sound often triggered a definite reaction. Whenever the telephone rang he would tell his owner, ***"Zei nisht a nar*** [Don't be a fool]." ***"Enfer dus!*** [Answer it!]"

• In Massachusetts, a yellow-faced rainbow blue budgerigar had his own private telephone listing, and when he was in a receptive mood his owner would hold the phone and he'd answer. But if he was indisposed his understanding owner simply said, "Master Yarrow prefers not to be disturbed. Do ring back tomorrow."

• A white cockatoo belonging to comedian Red Skelton possessed an uncanny record of being able to predict the future. One of the bird's outstanding feats was to warn the television star of the impending and untimely death of Skelton's close friend, Gene Fowler. On Fowler's last visit to the Skelton home there was no mistaking the look on the bird's face as she gazed at the Hollywood writer. The cockatoo was usually a happy creature, but during this visit she was totally silent and refused to remove her sad-looking eyes from Fowler's face.

• An Indian Hill mynah bird who resides in southern California earned more than $1,000 last year by singing and telling jokes at nightclubs and children's parties. The bird has a hefty bank account drawn up in his own name: Knight Lancelot III.

• A parrot living in Missouri often delivers a condensed version of the theory of relativity and can also recite other intricate formulas, including one for making nylon. The owner, a distinguished chemical engineer, often tried to disconcert the bird, but the parrot refused to be tricked. I watched the bird vigorously shake his head from side to side and stick to the correct rendition.

I talked to many scientists who feel that, of all the animals in the world, they have the greatest chance of obtaining non-human communication data by closely watching birds. This may be because some birds are the only animals who can successfully imitate human speech. Whatever the reason, the scientists said, many birds tend to be exhibitionists and allow their sounds and gestures to be easily observed.

Birds interact and respond to each other, and when this happens there is often an exchange of signals—these make up the language. Both visual and oral signals are used for communication, and, unlike dogs and cats, birds do not depend on facial expressions to reveal their thoughts.

Although there is no standard set of signals, many birds master between fifteen and thirty-five vocal and visual signals. Black-capped chickadees are said to have sixteen, the song sparrow is reported to have twenty-one, and the greater titmouse is supposed to possess at least thirty-five.

Scientists are busy interpreting them. In the Department of Ornithology at Cornell University, thirteen scientists have received grants from the National Science Foundation and the National Institutes of Health to conduct comparative ethological studies. Many other institutions of higher learning also have special departments that are devoted solely to the study of birds. Among them are Penn State, Purdue, Wisconsin, and Iowa State.

Dr. Konrad Lorenz, who is considered the father of the science of ethology—the study of the behavior of animals—has been "talking" to birds for a long time. Dr.

Lorenz, whom Julian Huxley calls, "one of the out-standing naturalists of our day," is a very, very cautious scientist and rarely issues positive-sounding statements, yet he has said, "The sentimental animal owner will often credit the bird with human intelligence. This is of course incorrect ... *but I do think that some birds possess a complicated code of signals which can be understood*" (italics mine).

Often the "understanding" may take many months of patient observation, but many bird owners told me that after a relatively brief period—days or weeks—of close observation they were not only able to interpret the true meaning of their bird's songs and movements, but were able to make the bird understand human actions as well.

For centuries man has been intrigued with bird songs and has thought that they merely indicated that the winged creatures were exhibiting great joy. They also felt that the song patterns were hereditary. Now these suppositions are subjects of grave doubt. Experiments seem to indicate that bird songs are learned. When birds have been raised far away from their own kind they are not able to reproduce songs considered typical to the breed. Left alone, such birds would never be able to mate or even fend for themselves because bird songs are not only important in mating but also in many other bird activities. Recently, scientists have discovered that most of the songs are part of a bird's complex communication system and that they convey information about courtship, mating, flight, weather, fear, and identification.

When sexually aroused, birds have special songs. While singing them, they often leap high into the air, or dance furiously and work themselves up to feverish pitch. The birds seem to be saying, "**Am I not superior to all others?**"

The scientists learned that the female wren emits a ringing squeal, the flicker makes a loud cry, and the male cowbird utters a shrill descending chirp when they actively seek mates. The food call may consist of a hoarse reprimand to a forgetful owner. The bird may be telling him, "**It's late, where's my food?**"

The nightingale's "**whip-poor-will,**" which is warbled continuously, often helps protect the bird from enemies. He seems to be warning others, "**I'm a pretty tough bird—stay away!**"

The precise details of the "language" differ for every species, but definite semantic clues can be picked up by an alert owner. Here are some owners who did.

First Lady of Birdland

Miriam Johnson, of Wilmington, Delaware, is accustomed to her alias and promptly responds to it. "I guess it was more frequent," she told me proudly, "when Lyndon Johnson and his wife, Lady Bird, were occupying the White House, but even now I often get called 'Bird Lady' Johnson. I don't object. Why spoil people's fun? After all, my husband and I do own birds!"

She and her husband, William, have kept a large variety of birds ever since they were married forty-three years ago. Mr. Johnson is a retired pharmacist, and his wife said, "Thank God Bill knows a great deal about doctoring birds. I guess he learned it from years behind the prescription counter." Then she added, with hauteur, "I'm sure Bill knows more about taking care of the sick than a lot of doctors!"

I talked to "Bird Lady" Johnson in her small, fiveroom stucco house, which could have been used as the illustration for the fairytale story of the gingerbread house. Because six birds were in constant residence, it appeared even smaller. Yet it possessed a great deal of charm and despite its use as an aviary it was one of the most immaculate houses I've ever been in.

Miriam Johnson: "Currently we have six birds living with us, or I should say we are living with them! There's Millie, who is a scarlet macaw; Lennie, a yellow canary; Arkie, a zebra finch; a pair of Madagascar lovebirds, named Frankie and Johnnie; and . . . whatever is the name of the other bird? I just can't remember—for the life of me I can't remember! Oh, yes, it's coming to me. How could I forget Donnie, our sulphur-crested cockatoo?

"At one time, Bill and I had lots more, but Bill says now that six is more than enough. Actually, birds don't require much taking care of. We travel a great deal these days, and I get a bird-sitter to tend them. Oh, I'm very careful to get someone who really loves birds. It isn't enough to say you do—a body has to feel that way deep down. We have a nice young high school senior who takes care of them while we're away. She's a pure gem! I've discovered that age has nothing to do with responsibility.

"As a matter of fact, our young sitter has intently scrutinized the birds and reported some interesting facts to us: when something uncomfortable occurred to the lovebirds, the direction of their feathers often reflected their moods—feathers pointing down usually meant they were saying, 'Things are real tough!' Feathers up meant, 'Things are okay!'

"When the canary held his head to the right side and stuck his neck far out he usually warbled a song that meant, 'Come and be sociable.' And when the macaw preens, it may mean she's nervous because it's often followed by sweating.

"Millie, the macaw, is a big one—over three feet tall. Why, if she wanted to I suppose her beak is powerful enough to bite right out of her cage. But she doesn't—she knows how we feel about her and so she's very devoted to us. Lennie, our canary, is a joy to behold and such a comfort. He, too, knows us well—we make it a point to communicate love and tenderness to all the birds. Lennie sings a good morning song the moment we go near him at the start of the day. When I came down recently with a severe case of pneumonia and was confined to bed for weeks, Bill moved Lennie's cage into the bedroom. Lennie comforted me by singing all day long—he knew how appreciative I was. I'd clap my hands afer each rendition and offer great praise. Lennie loves bits of dog biscuits and I often reward him with a tiny sliver. He was so appreciative.

"Then we come to Arkie. He's about the size of my hand and, for laughs, I often put him alongside giant Millie—they look like Mutt and Jeff. Arkie has a black and white chest, an orange beak, and orange legs. I could watch him for hours—he always puts on a show. He dotes on praise and I'm careful to tell him how great I think he is. He can recognize praise and when I compliment him his chest really puffs out and he begins to strut. I've trained him to sit on my pinky finger, but Bill has gone me one better—he has taught Arkie to sit on the very tip of his nose.

"Frankie and Johnnie are our two lovebirds, but we have learned to keep them away from the other birds. At times they're too sassy for their own good and then we separate them from each other, too. But then they say that true love isn't always smooth. It sure isn't in their case.

"They know when I scold them. I'll raise my voice almost to a shout and say firmly, 'You have both been very naughty! I'm ashamed of you!' They'll lower their heads as if they're repenting, and for the next few hours or days they behave real well toward me and each other. They're excellent breeders and we have sold many of their offspring.

"Then we come to . . . I forgot again. If Bill were here he'd say that there must be something real Freudian about my constant forgetting. How can I possibly leave Donnie out? He's truly my pride and joy! He's also large, but not quite as huge as Millie. Donnie doesn't talk frequently, but when he does it proves how intelligent he is. If he were a student attending public school I'm sure he'd lead the class. Donnie's been with us for a long time—going on twenty-two years in February, and I feel he'll be around for another twenty. I'm certain of one thing: he'll survive us. I'm sixty-eight now, but I honestly think the birds keep me feeling younger. Who knows, we may be around to celebrate his forty-second birthday!"

"Birds Are God's Gift to Man . . . and Woman"

Henry Spellman plans on getting married next June. "Don't think it was easy," he told me. "My intended's mother had real doubts about me as a son-in-law. She told Laura, her daughter, that I was the type that's a confirmed bachelor—that at the ripe old age of thirty-eight I was used to living alone and that I was set in my ways. Then she'd add the clincher: 'What man,' she'd say, 'would keep a bird? I ask you? There has to be something wrong with him!' "

Fortunately for Henry, Laura likes birds and has blissfully agreed to the marriage. She has also assented to take the bird—a two-year-old albino parakeet—into their new home in northern New Jersey. But what's completed Henry's happiness is that Laura's mother finally met the parakeet, fell in love with him, and promptly bought an almost exact duplicate.

Henry has a responsible, well-paying position as a cost accountant for a large insurance company. "I know it sounds dull," he said, "but some of my audits reveal such deviousness and require such ingenuity on my part that even Sam Spade, the private eye in fiction, would be envious."

Although Henry likes to cook, he also likes to bowl, water ski, and dance. At college he played center on the junior varsity team, which is how his nose got broken. He likes children and plans on having several of them. "After all," he told me, "if I can take care of a parakeet, I certainly can handle human creatures!"

Henry Spellman: "I think what really sold my future mother-in-law on birds was a true story I told her. It seems that a man named Sam Geller owned a restaurant called the Green Parrot in honor of his very clever talking bird. One evening while tending bar Sam was fatally shot by a drunk who immediately fled.

"Police promptly investigated and could only find one clue: the parrot kept repeating, '**Robert! Robert!**' There were a lot of Roberts who visited the Green Parrot, and the police visited them all. With the exception of one, all were able to furnish satisfactory alibis. One Robert had vanished from the neighborhood and the police couldn't locate him, but about a year later the police learned his whereabouts and picked him up. This Robert promptly admitted the crime and said, 'That bird is too damn smart! I never liked him and now I know why!' Robert was sentenced to Sing Sing prison.

"Soon after I finished the tale, Laura's mother assented to my marriage and promptly went out to buy a talking bird. We kid about it now, but she agrees that the 'green parrot' was a very fascinating bird commentary.

"Now that she, too, is a bird owner she suddenly regards me as a great ornithologist and constantly seeks my counsel. I must admit I like the role of being a bird authority. But the truth be known, I've given her some very sound advice that will help her to communicate with her bird. One of the first things I told her was to put the bird's cage in a place where he will have frequent human company. In this way the bird will become accustomed to regular companionship and will realize that no one intends to harm him.

"I always stand close to my bird's head when I'm training him. I repeat each word slowly, perhaps ten or fifteen times. I do not make any sudden move, because if you do, the bird will surely be frightened and, from then on, any future lesson could prove fruitless. For best teaching results I darken the room and make sure the radio or television is turned off—*this is one time you don't want competition!*

"Do not try to teach the bird too large a vocabulary in the beginning—concentrate on a few words a day. The length of the session should be kept brief—not more than fifteen minutes—because I've found that birds lose interest rapidly. I've also discovered that in the beginning it's best to use words that end in vowel sounds: *lovely, pretty, bye-bye.* The pitch of your voice is very important—raise it several octaves above normal.

"Many bird owners have told me that their pets are very sensitive to barometric pressure changes. I've found this is true, because my birds reacts strongly to all meteorological vibrations. Often, I can determine weather changes merely by closely observing his movements.

"Another thing is that birds will miss you when you're away for a long time. They develop all kinds of strange symptoms and then go downhill in a hurry. Once I had to make a company trip to England, and when I returned I was told that my bird had developed a tumor. I knew that parakeets frequently came down with tumors, but fortunately this one turned out to be psychosomatic.

"Everybody has an embarrassing story concerning swearing and their 'talking' bird. Mine occurred when the vice-president of my firm and his very straight-laced wife visited me—and the bird let out with a long string of four-letter words. Since that time I've been extra careful about swearing in the bird's presence. My theory is that birds pick up swear words easily because they're usually uttered with such great emphasis.

"Perhaps it's because of that fact that birds seem so very human and it constantly amazes me how they can perform such Herculean tasks. Bower birds in Australia actually paint the walls of their shelters with fruit pulp and with paste of chewed-up grass mixed with saliva. Then they decorate them with colored glass and shells. While this is going on, they chirp a merry tune that sounds like, '**Pretty house. Pretty house.**'

"Their performance makes me think of a poem I learned when I was in the fifth or sixth grade—it was by Henry Wadsworth Longfellow and I had to memorize it:

"Learned of every bird its language
"Learned their names and all their secrets,
"Talked with them whenever we met them."

Two questions are asked all the time: "Can a bird—talking or otherwise—be trained? And once trained, does he really *understand* what he's being taught?"

Bird owners responded to both queries with an unqualified "Yes!" They revealed how they have succeeded in teaching their pet to beg, to play dead, and even say prayers.

"My mynah knows what I ask for," said Carol Abrams of Albany, New York. "I purposely try to cross her up, but she's too smart for any of my trickery."

I was told about an aviary at the Busch Gardens in St. Louis where, several times a day, viewers watch a large-crested cockatoo push a toy cart with his beak, and they marvel as a powerful-looking macaw seizes a ring with his beak and slides down a seventy-five-foot wire. Whenever the birds and the trainer feel that the performances are below par the birds quickly try again.

Dr. Malcolm Noyes, an English psychologist, says, "Most birds can be trained if the owner has sufficient patience and is prepared to offer an instantaneous reward. It doesn't do to give compensation moments after the act has been accomplished—even a slight delay will prove ineffectual. To get positive results one has to act rapidly. The results are most worthwhile. My Lady Gould finch loves tiny bits of peeled apple. She stands on her head and rolls over and over to get some."

CHAPTER X

How Pets Can Communicate through ESP

Most pets hate baths and will take to their heels at the first whiff of a cake of flea soap. Some learn to recognize the meaning of the word *bath*, or even its spelling. But Bachelor Bill, a cocker spaniel we once owned, was more sensitive than that. We needed only to begin thinking about giving that dog a bath and he would cock his ears, close his eyes, start howling, and vanish under the front porch for the rest of the day. Was he psychic? Did he possess some uncanny sixth sense and was he able to read our minds?

Some doubters would explain it away by saying that the dog was responding to an unconscious vocal tone or facial expression on the part of the human who was bent on dog-washing. Perhaps so. Yet many puzzled pet owners report far more uncanny performances by so-called dumb beasts every year.

A dog howls miserably all night—and next morning the family learns that his absent master is dead. A surplus cat, bundled in a sack, is hauled fifty miles out of town and dumped on a lonely road, but is back on the doorstep two days later. A pet bird suddenly refuses to eat because his vacationing mistress—five hundred miles away—has become ill. Other inexplicable relationships between humans and animals are frequently reported.

What strange power of communication is at work?

Many outstanding scientists and investigators now accept the idea that some human beings can communicate with one another by telepathy and are able to acquire all kinds of mysterious information by means of extrasensory perception. *These researchers are discovering that household pets may be superior to humans and very often communicate by telepathy.*

This may be the answer to such intriguing questions as:

• How does a dog—or cat—know that his master will enter the house in five minutes, even though the owner comes home each day at different times?

• How does a bird know several days in advance of an impending cyclone and try desperately to break out of his cage and fly to safety?

Animals seem to possess senses that man has lost or never had . . . see sights that humans shall never see . . . hear sounds man shall never hear. Today, the psychic abilities of household pets are the subject of exciting new research by parapsychologists—specialists in ESP.

The body of documented evidence begins with the famous case of Ignace Paderewski's parrot. In his writings, the great musician and premier of Poland said that the bird's harsh, scratchy voice grated on his nerves, yet Cocky Roberts was for many years his devoted pet. Friends tell how the bird would tap on the door of Paderewski's study with his beak, screaming, "**This is Cocky Roberts! Let me in!**"

Years later, when the aging bird had been given into the care of a friend in Switzerland, Paderewski, asleep in a New York City hotel room, heard the parrot's voice in his dreams. It was screeching piteously, "**This is Cocky Roberts! Let me in!**" The musician awoke with the conviction that his pet was dead. About a week later he received a letter saying that on the night of his dream the parrot, in perfect health, had been accidentally shut out of the house on a bitterly cold night and had frozen to death on the doorstep.

A similar story—but with a happy ending—was reported by a Toledo, Ohio, accountant who awoke with a sudden start one night, convinced that his dog was racing frantically around the bedroom. The room was empty. He went to the dog's usual sleeping place and found the animal unconscious, tangled in its leash and nearly choked to death. There is no doubt that the dream, or half-waking impression, saved the dog's life.

Human-to-animal telepathy was the subject of a prolonged laboratory experiment with six kittens by Dr. Karlis Osis, a parapsychologist working under a Rockefeller Foundation grant at Duke University. Dr. Osis and his aides built an eighteen-foot-long, tube-like passageway with several right-angle turns in it. At the end there were two metal cups containing cat food.

One by one, the kittens were released into the passageway while the experimenter, sitting behind a screen, concentrated on mentally urging the animal to choose one of the two cups.

In all, 3,900 trials were conducted. The feline responses should have been so-so, yet the kittens responded far above the chance level, which indicated that perhaps ESP accounted for the increase. (The experimenters were careful to mask all odors.) Most exciting was the outstanding performance of a striped kitty named Judy, who selected the "right" cup as much as 50 percent above chance. This and other experiments have convinced Dr. Osis that an alert owner can constructively use ESP with his animal.

One owner had trained Pikki, his fox terrier, to make constant use of telepathy. Pikki was the star of a famous European dog act witnessed by thousands. The dog's trainer could stand behind a thick screen or even in another room and, silent and unseen, give commands that the dog obeyed instantly. The dog's uncanny communication came to the attention of the academic world and Dr. W. Bechterev, a Russian neurologist, was sent to investigate. After administering a battery of tests, Dr. Bechterev found that he, too, could order the dog around simply by picturing what he wanted done and giving the mental command, "Go!" Other scientists reported similar results.

The Pikki incident is one of many that appear in the files of the Parapsychology Laboratory of Duke University, headed by Dr. J. B. Rhine. Another case that received great attention was that of a collie whose owner was the superintendent of a large explosives plant. One day the man appeared at the plant without the dog, who had always accompanied him on his walk to work. He explained that he and the collie had left the house together that morning as usual, but when they drew near the plant area the dog started to whine piteously, sat down on the ground and, although he was usually very obedient, refused to move. Impatiently, the man had gone to work and left the animal sitting there. When he arrived in his office he found an anxious telephone message from his wife, saying the collie had returned home and was panting, whining, and trembling beneath their bed.

The morning was uneventful and at noon the superintendent went out to lunch. When he finished, he returned to the plant. *Half an hour later the entire factory blew up, killing many employees—including the collie's master!*

If the superintendent had been able to understand the dog's urgent message could the tragedy have been averted? Parapsychologists are trying to find out. They realize that the man or woman who can make willful, voluntary use of ESP powers is still comparatively rare. But they are discovering that a "sixth sense," unusual to most humans, may be ever-present in dogs, cats, and birds.

"What is needed," said Dr. Osis, "is an informed owner. Man has to learn to understand animal ESP and learn to make it work constructively."

A remarkable incident that reveals an animal's psychic communicating powers concerns Shep, a Scotch shepherd dog, and his owner, Francis McMahon of Rock Island, Illinois. McMahon had to go down to his basement to make some minor repairs. The dog, usually very quiet, started to bark loudly. McMahon patted him and entered the cellar. He slipped on the steps and was immediately carted off to a nearby hospital. The dog followed, and before McMahon's stretcher was moved into the emergency room he managed to whisper to Shep, "Don't worry. It'll be all right. I'll come back after they fix me up. Wait for me here!"

The occurrence took place in the lobby of the hospital. Shep knew exactly what his master had told him and waited patiently, but McMahon never returned —he died of complications of a severe skull fracture. Shep didn't see the body as it was removed through the rear exit, a great distance away from the dog. Many soundproof doors separated the dog from the rear exit.

A hospital orderly reported: "Shep was usually very quiet, but that moment he started barking furiously. I honestly think Shep knew that something terrible had happened to his master, but he was told to wait—and wait he did. I swear that dog was saying, '**I was told to remain right here!**' "

The Franciscan sisters who ran the hospital provided Shep with food, and for twelve years the dog waited in vain for his master. Only Shep's death ended the strange vigil. The American Humane Association was made aware of the dog's devotion to a spoken message and erected a plaque in the hospital lobby where Shep had waited so many years—because his owner had told him to.

Some years ago the entire nation was thrilled by the feat of another dog. Bobbie was owned by an Oregon family named Brazier who were driving east on a vacation when Bobbie jumped out of their car near

Wolcott, Indiana, to join a dog fight. Somehow the family didn't realize the dog had left until it was too late. They continued their journey and drove home several weeks later via Mexico.

Six months later, thin and exhausted, Bobbie turned up in the Braziers' front yard in Oregon. Affidavits by Humane Societies and other evidence showed that Bobbie did not return the way he had come. Nor did he trail the family home through Mexico. Instead, he'd turned around, crossed the Rockies, and headed straight for the Northwest coast!

Clementine, an equally remarkable seven-toed cat, was left behind when her owners moved from New York to Colorado. Clementine was about to have kittens. She raised the litter, weaned them, and they disappeared. Three months later she walked triumphantly through the kitchen door of her owners' new home in Denver—1,795 miles away! Clementine was nearly starved and her paws were cracked and bleeding, but it was unmistakably the same cat.

Dr. Rhine and his associates rule out cases that lack positive identifying marks. One black eye or a furry tail is not unique. So one important criterion is that the pet possess some clearly identifiable mark. Many other alleged telepathy cases are ruled out because the animal started out from a place not too far away and could have reached its goal by random wandering or spiral circling until a familiar scent was picked up.

The most familiar animal that "homes" instinctively is the carrier pigeon. During World War I, a French carrier pigeon earned fame by transmitting important messages across enemy lines, undaunted by murderous gunfire. Traditionally, homing pigeons are taught to return to their roost by exposure to repeated training trips—each trip is a little farther away from home.

Up until 1949, it had been assumed that pigeons find their way by whirling around in the air until they sight a familiar landmark. But in that year, Dr. G. V. T. Matthews, an English zoologist, gathered a group of twenty-five pigeons and trained them to "home" from the north. When they were well trained —up to 125 miles—Dr. Matthews put them in a truck in cloth-draped cages and carted them eighty miles west. He released them and they promptly flew straight home. He took them ninety miles south—with the same result.

Dr. Matthews' discovery has been widely put to use and today the United States Air Force is assigning pigeons to help pilot planes. The air force of the Soviet Union recently credited a pigeon with *guiding a lost plane through thick clouds right onto a runway.*

"Of course," we might say, "not all animals show startling talent at finding their way home. After all, many pets wander off each day and are never seen again." But we don't know whether they all want to return. We don't know whether they can turn their homing talents on and off at will. Scientists have not yet penetrated the complex machinery of the nervous system which enables animals to perform these incredible feats.

Yet, as we have seen, there is impressive authenticated, spontaneous evidence and careful laboratory research that seems to show that animals can communicate with the human world. Can we learn valuable ESP secrets from our pets? Many scientists to whom I talked think so, and with the experiments now going on in parapsychology laboratories, we may very soon discover that the dog, cat, or bird in your home possesses a high degree of ESP—and can literally read your mind.

"However, far more important for you, the owner," said Dr. Eugene Cushman, a California psychologist, "is the fact that this is one more way in which you and your pet can communicate." Dr. Cushman, who has conducted dozens of ESP experiments, added, "There is an easy way to determine the amount of ESP your pet has—and that is to observe him. Not just for one day, or for two days, but for many days. Look and listen carefully. Armed with this knowledge you will know when he's trying to tell you something."

I asked many of the scientists engaged in animal communication projects why they were spending money, time, and effort on experiments that some people might regard as frivolous. Dr. Borgese, the California animal behaviorist, put her reply this way:

"If these experiments can make even the tiniest contribution to the understanding of linguistic behavior and learning in animals and to the possibility of communicating with them, the effort will have been well worthwhile ... for [animal] language is the gateway to the future."

A major breakthrough in pet communication seems imminent. Animal behaviorists expect it to happen within the next decade and offer the following reasons for the importance of this event:

- With the increased population having to occupy limited space, scientists are eager to learn the secret of why pets manage to live harmoniously in small —sometimes incredibly small—areas. This doesn't mean that the scientists expect animals to suddenly start discussing their living conditions in rich prose; but, by understanding and interpreting animal language, we will be able to know what elements in their environments make them satisfied or unhappy—and also why.

- Currently, there are large groups of men, women, and children who find it difficult to—or simply can't —communicate. Researchers feel that animals can help tremendously in teaching us how to help these unfortunate human beings by showing us ways to communicate with less than normal human methods—fewer skills, less physiological and brain equipment, and perhaps a different order of priorities.

- With pet-bites on the rise, we want to be able to read an animal's language accurately so that we will know when he's aroused, angry, or afraid. Some school authorities are even now considering a new basic course in pet communication for students in lower grades so that the incidence of bites might be reduced.

- Animal behaviorists are certain that through language we will be able to achieve a greater accord and understanding in living with our pets. And we will finally discover how much they know, how much they can learn, and how much they can communicate if we will give them the chance they deserve.

Does that mean that in ten or twenty years we can expect pet owners to carry on long, involved philosophical conversations with their animals or have the pets make unreasonable demands like insisting on vacations in Florida and skiing trips to Vermont? Does it mean that Clifford Simak's science-fiction novel *City* will actually happen, that—just as in the book—dogs will take over from ineffective man and rule the world?

"NO!" is my emphatic answer. No amount of training will turn your pet into a being remotely as intelligent as a human. If that's what you have in mind, don't try. But if your goal is a happier animal and a happier owner, I suggest that you do start learning how to converse with your pet. You will be delighted with the results!

CHAPTER XI

How Horses Communicate

Most people rightly don't consider horses household pets, although my two daughters always wanted to bring their twelve-hundred-pound animals into the kitchen and feed them hot oats and turnips. The fact is, nevertheless, that most horses object to being domesticated. Everybody knows that they don't cuddle like cats; nor are they protective like dogs. Most of them rarely make joyful sounds like birds. Scientists who have carefully studied horses tells us that their intelligence is limited; that they often do not appear to be particularly grateful for food, shelter or grooming; that they are not known for such heroics as attempts to save their masters' lives.

One Harvard psychologist told me, "A horse will suddenly stop short on a river bank, pitch its rider into the water, calmly eat grass and then trot back to his stable while the owner struggles in the current or floats downstream. If a horse drags his injured owner home, you can be pretty sure it's because the rider's foot is caught in the stirrup. Anyone who believes romanticized stories that say otherwise has never observed horses carefully!"

Regardless of these sober and negative views, some 300,000 horses in the United States are considered "pets"—which is to say that they (and often their families) live in a state of interrelationship with human families and are dependent on these owners. Happily, I'm included in that number, and after interviewing dozens of scientists, trainers, successful owners and others close to horses, I have reaffirmed a long-standing conviction of mine: if you will just give this great, powerful four-legged friend and servant a chance, he will prove to you that he is the most versatile of animals—if not one of the most communicative. Again and again I was told that a horse quickly adapts himself to his environment and has a superb memory.

The communicating signals of a horse may not be as numerous as those of a cat or dog, but I believe that an observant owner can readily learn to understand what a horse is saying. The late British Colonel Charles E. G. Hope, formerly of the Indian Cavalry and recognized throughout the riding world as an outstanding equestrian authority, said, "A horse is a very emotional and willing being, who at frequent intervals wants to understand and be understood, but the bloody trick is learning how. . . . It isn't too difficult to accomplish—if you know what to look for and don't expect great miracles. *Remember, even though the horse's comprehension exists, it is limited.*" (Italics mine.)

Teddy Wahl, owner of the Round Hill Stable in Greenwich, Connecticut, believes that horses produce a lot more communication signals than most humans are alert enough to interpret. He says, "A horse will signal with his voice, ears, tail and with other parts of his body. In the stall, for example, he flattens you against the wall if he doesn't like what you're doing—such as grooming a tangled mane or applying medication to a lame foot. He's not just moving out of the way; he is plainly telling you to get lost."

Wahl, who has worked with horses for more than fifty years, adds, "The main source of communication between rider and horse is mind and muscle. What's in the rider's mind is communicated to the horse through the rider's body movement, tension and relaxation. If you make a sudden grab of the reins and jab the horse in the mouth, you'll naturally have a scared, unsteady horse and a very bad ride. Put your mind on the consequences of your communications. Think ahead: what's likely to be coming up over the fence and around the turn? But try never to think scared or negative or helpless—like 'What'll I do if he doesn't . . . ?' "

Many people who don't know horses presume that the extent of their comprehension of the human voice is "Whoah!" Informed owners strongly disagree. They know that the horse's knowledge is infinitely greater, and with proper training he can easily distinguish oral commands, the most basic ones being "*Walk, trot, canter.*"

Animal behaviorists add that a great deal of what a horse understands depends on the tone of the human voice. *Walk* and *trot,* the experts say, may contain an equal number of letters, but *trot* is usually delivered more forcefully and *canter* even more so. The experts have discovered that owners who raise their voices ever-so-slightly and speak in a calm and a reasonable manner get the best results. Speaking with a Southern accent or Western drawl gets best results. The scientists have also found that the horse, more than most animals, refuses to "converse" whenever he is under the slightest threat of punishment.

Dr. F. Dudley Klopfer, professor of psychology at Washington State University, told me, "The horse is a highly trained animal, but does not give up its vices under the application of strongly adversive stimulation such as whipping or scolding, but withdraws instead."

Parapsychologists, who know about ESP, go further. They feel that under such circumstances the horse will frequently call on his "sixth sense" and "psych" himself out of his predicament.

I heard of many such incidents, including one that had recently occurred near Cambridge, Massachusetts, where Lem, an unusually mild-mannered Shetland pony, resorted to ESP to alleviate what he considered intolerable conditions of his life. Specifically, Lem was being persistently berated.

"I was asleep," his precocious twelve-year-old owner said. "Suddenly, Lem appeared in my dream. I guess it was more of a *nightmare*. Get it? *Night! Mare!* He spoke to me clear as day. 'I've had enough of your temper!' he told me. 'I'm leaving!' Quick like a bunny, I ran to the stable and, sure enough, Lem had broken out of his stall and was trying to kick down part of the pasture fence. If I hadn't arrived right then I'm sure he would have done it." The girl's father, who had accompanied his daughter that night, corroborated everything she said.

Most academicians to whom I talked about ESP between horses and humans were doubtful, at least for the present. Most of them said, "I suppose it's possible, but ... " I found it difficult to get further into this subject because little accepted research exists on horse clairvoyance or telepathy. Yet many owners had an ESP tale to relate about "man's greatest servant."

How Horses Communicate

The most famous case of a psychic horse occurred in Germany at the turn of the century. At that time stories began circulating about Hans, a stallion, who gave correct answers to mathematical problems. For example, when the horse was asked by its owner, Herr Wilhelm von Osten, a retired schoolteacher, to add three plus three, Hans would immediately paw the ground and stamp his left hoof six times. Four and four got eight hoof taps. "Clever Hans," as the horse was soon called, also excelled in multiplication and division. Before long his repertoire included fractions and cube roots.

Clever Hans' fame spread throughout Europe. A group of distinguished scientists visited him and reported that he "possessed a great intellect made possible through psychic ability." Soon, other scientists arrived at his stable in Berlin for further observations, and most of their findings were similar to the first: "Clever Hans is truly an equine genius!"

One academician, however, noticed that Clever Hans failed to answer correctly whenever von Osten wasn't clearly visible. This suggested that perhaps the owner, a highly reputable and honorable man, was unconsciously supplying the horse with answers. Further tests bore out this theory. Whenever the horse pawed the ground the proper number of times, the owner, who had solved the problem in his head, looked relieved and relaxed slightly. These unintended signals were clear enough for Hans to detect and he immediately concluded that it was time to stop. Von Osten was publicly disgraced and soon died of a broken heart, but even his most severe critics had to admit that Hans was clever enough to pick up signals that were all but invisible.

Another memorable ESP case history took place in the Russian Cavalry during World War II. There is at least one documented instance of Soviet mounted troops advancing rapidly and being forced to cross a heavily mined battlefield. Records show that the riders who allowed their horses to find their own way got through unscathed, but the Cavalry soldiers who insisted on guiding their mounts were instantly blown up.

Most riders with whom I talked accepted the old folk saying that insists, "Drop the reins and he'll take you home." They told me dozens of "lost-with-a-horse" stories to demonstrate the saying's veracity.

Does all this prove that horses possess a sixth sense? We will have to wait a bit longer to find out. Soviet researchers are presently conducting a series of ESP experiments with horses, but they won't make the results known for several years.

Authorities told me that there is little doubt that a horse knows when a human is fearful or uncertain. June Reno, a former U.S. Pony Club District Commissioner, says: "If you enter a stall carrying the bridle and think, 'Oh, dear, he's going to give me trouble and I'll never get the bridle on'—then you won't! Sure, a horse will occasionally bolt or do something completely opposite to your commands. That's usually because you've failed to communicate your wishes properly, but you've done all too well communicating your fears."

The late Colonel Charles Hope shared the same view: "Perhaps, when a horse fails to translate the human language correctly, he is not just a bloody fool, but has not been given the signals correctly. Like the computer when it is given the wrong program, it [the horse] becomes confused, which makes it frightened and obstinate, and finally violent."

When it's the rider's turn to receive messages from the horse, the animal is usually very precise in delivering them. Although their significance may differ somewhat from those of a stablemate, there is a surprisingly wide variety of signs that most horses use to convey thoughts. Some of the most frequent ones will be found in the Pet Communication Dictionary.

CHAPTER XII

Do's and Don'ts for Effective Pet Communication

You have just received loads of practical advice on how to carry on effective two-way conversations with your pet. Academicians, veterinarians, trainers, and other professionals who work with animals have provided explicit details. You have also heard perceptive owners explain their communication triumphs in simple terms, without resorting to scientific jargon, illustrating their remarks with personal experiences. All these men and women acknowledge that they occasionally encounter roadblocks. In this section I've collected some tips to help you get around these problems.

While most of these do's and don'ts apply equally to dogs and cats (less so to birds and horses) you may think that some solutions are not applicable to your particular pet. Regardless, I commend these points to your attention because an irrelevant suggestion might suddenly trigger a relevant one, or you may discover that a combination of two or more solutions will work wonders in your own situation.

Remember, too, that all these do's and don'ts have been included because they have been found useful for animal communication; these are not whimsical creations of impractical people who are far removed from animals—they see and work with them every day. So the next time your pet appears lackadaisical or refuses to cooperate, look to this list for help.

Do's

1. **Do be realistic** and set a goal that an animal can be reasonably expected to accomplish. It's foolish to presume that a very tiny Pekingese will be able to fetch the bulky Sunday *Times* or that a silver tabby will be able to recite the Gettysburg Address.

2. **Do watch the tone of your voice.** Pitch it slightly higher than usual since most pets seem to understand you better when it is raised. But don't make the error once committed by the late Tallulah Bankhead. The actress had been asked by a friend to look after his cat while he was touring in England. She assented and agreed to all his advice, which included speaking to the cat in a "sweet tone." Ms. Bankhead was known for her deep, throaty voice and purposely raised it several octaves every time she spoke to the animal. But each time she tried, the cat seemed puzzled. Ms. Bankhead's reaction was to increase her volume, rather than her pitch. Soon she was shouting so ferociously that the

actress' startled neighbors rushed in to protect her from invaders.

3. Do say things as if you mean them. Some authorities feel that the animal only recognizes the tone of voice and responds accordingly. Others told me that key words triggered the action. And still others claimed that pets could recognize most words. All agreed, however, that the tone of voice was all important. A soft, questioning tone will not make Tabby refrain from dangling out the open window; a gruff shout won't encourage Fido to lick your hand. It isn't efficient to say "nice" things in a "nasty" tone in order to stimulate your pet into action.

4. Do speak distinctly. Occasionally, listen to yourself; a tape recorder is an excellent device for this rehearsal purpose. Remember, enunciate clearly and go s-l-o-w-l-y.

5. Do repeat. All the animal behaviorists and owners insisted that this *do* is very significant. Some words and phrases have to be reiterated over and over and over before comprehension begins. You may become weary of the constant repetition, but your pet rarely will.

6. Do use simple, one-syllable words at first, such as: *food, ball, run, chair, hat.* It's fun to have the pet recognize "antidisestablishmentarianism"—but that's all it is, a stunt, hardly very practical conversational material.

7. **Do keep on talking and don't give up.** I found that the best and most meaningful two-way conversation existed when the owner spoke to the pet constantly. Not a lot of gibberish, but often just light-hearted talk like, "That's a lovely sky," or "The refrigerator needs defrosting," will condition a pet to the idea of becoming a conversational partner, and this can eventually produce amazing results. You'll be surprised and pleased to notice how much the animal picks up from these frivolous chats as time—and talk—flows by.

8. **Do play with your pet.** They all enjoy periods of not-too-rough rough-house games. It won't work to say that you haven't the time. Theodore Roosevelt was a very busy man, yet he romped with his animals each evening. Both they and the president loved it.

9. **Do see the world from the pet's vantage point.** It's important to bear in mind that most things appear huge and wondrous to an animal. Discover what his world looks like by occasionally getting down on all fours.

10. **Do use common sense.** Many of your communication problems can be solved by applying just old-fashioned savvy or applying the same set of standards that you would with a child.

11. **Do always make sure that your pet has been let out before you attempt to teach.** If you don't, he just can't keep his mind on his lessons. Could you?

12. **Do have the room quiet when you're working**

with your pet. Few people—and animals—can communicate very effectively in a noisy room. Turn the TV and radio off. Avoid constant interruptions.

13. **Do be observant.** This is another crucially important *do*, as I've stressed all along. Every movement your pet makes signifies something and has a special meaning. Learn what it is.

14. **Do compile a notebook when making your observations.** Even the best memory can benefit from a notebook. Keep one handy and start recording your pet's movements—and the apparent meanings. You'll soon be gratified at how helpful it will be.

15. **Do praise an animal often.** Verbal and non-verbal praise are equally essential. *Pet your pet.* Tell him that he's handsome. Tell him he's the finest animal in the whole world. And act as if you really mean it!

16. **Do let your pet know that you love him.** Animals, like children, have to be reassured again and again that they truly are loved. They enjoy hearing it and it costs you so little effort. Remember, both words and actions are necessary for the proper communication of love.

17. **Do respect the animal.** Albert Payson Terhune, the celebrated writer of dog stories, used to say: "Too many owners confuse love with respect or vice versa —they are not the same thing. If you invite the pet into your home, then he certainly should be worthy of some esteem."

18. **Do have patience.** You may think that your pet simply refuses to learn. The old axiom about trying again when you don't succeed applies doubly to animals. If you lack perseverance, this is a fine way to acquire some. If you refuse to keep trying, you surely will fail!

19. **Do try to follow the same daily routine.** Animals seem to love rituals and regard anything that is repeated daily as a delightful ceremony. Schedule your conversation lessons for the same hour each day. Give him the same reward. Pet him in a similar fashion. You may regard all this as dull stuff, but the animal will not.

20. **Do end each session on an upbeat note.** Give your pet some word or phrase that you are sure he's familiar with—that he has previously identified. Whenever you think he has responded properly, give him his reward and praise, and be generous about it. He will be so happy to come back for more the following day.

Don'ts

1. **Don't make any learning session too long.** Animals get exhausted easily and a fifteen-minute period should be sufficient. Sometimes your pet may prefer two shorter sessions. You have to play this by ear—his ear!

2. **Don't yell when he makes mistakes.** Be tolerant and allow him to fail occasionally. He may be trying, but simply doesn't yet get the hang of what's on your

mind. Most pets are extremely sensitive, and a great deal of harm can be done if you shout at errors. Remember: *sometimes even you make mistakes!*

3. Don't stop loving him because he makes mistakes. This doesn't mean that you have to be endlessly accepting of errors, but don't let your love be dependent on excellent performances either. Let him know that your love is constant, no matter what, even if you feel frustrated or annoyed from time to time.

4. Don't try to teach him when you're tired. If you do, you're likely to snap at a mediocre performance. Granted that a pet is conscious of your moods, but isn't it asking a little too much to have him forgive your irritability?

5. Don't be inconsistent. For instance, don't laugh at your pet's antics one day and frown upon them the next. Alvin Toffler, author of the bestselling book *Future Shock,* told me about one such incident. "We were amused," he said, "when our dog turned on the bathroom faucet when he wanted a drink. He was aware of our delight at his dexterity. But the dog couldn't turn the faucet off and the result was huge puddles of water. We finally had to be consistent and curb him of the faucet habit."

6. Don't reward your pet with things you *think* he likes, but with things you *know* he likes. I found some pets who hated animal biscuits, but just loved raw figs. It's easy to determine the likes and dislikes of your pet—he is very happy to demonstrate and even debate them.

7. **Don't use your voice alone.** As I've already emphasized, body movements also make language. This is one time when actions speak as loud as or louder than words. Get into the habit of using your face and body to accentuate something you're saying verbally. When you start out you should take extra care to be especially expressive.

8. **Don't say "No!" all the time.** A steady diet of "No" produces the obvious result—nothing. Your pet will get so used to your "No" that he may finally refuse to respond to any stimulus. Remember the story of the boy who cried "Wolf!" all the time? Reserve the negative verbal command for times you feel it's unquestionably necessary. This is a good time to reach for your notebook again. Record the number of times you say "No" and list the offenses they're used for. I'll bet they can be pruned way down.

9. **Don't be scared of your pet.** Too many owners are, and two-way communication rarely works when one of the partners is frightened of the other. (It works both ways—obviously, pets, too, can be alarmed by owners.)

10. **Don't lie to an animal.** Pets rarely tell falsehoods to you and they expect to be treated in similar fashion. If you tell him that you'll take him out if he does something properly, but you don't have any intention of doing it, this may work a few times, but soon the pet

will get wise—and then watch out. There are few places more frustrating than the receiving end of an animal's scorn.

11. Don't use baby talk. Speak to your pet as you would to a eight- or nine-year-old child. "*Oos ittle bitty kitty is oo?*" No "itchy-gitchy-goo" talk! Never!

12. Don't try to turn your pet into something he was never intended to be. Putting baby clothes on him won't help to make him human. He's a pet, first and always. But pets can be close friends.

13. Don't ask him to do something that you have no intention of seeing carried out. If the request is reasonable, see that he does it. You might say, "I want to sleep, stop making noise." If he continues being noisy, put him out of the room physically. Animal trainers told me that you will suffer serious setbacks if you don't back up your *reasonable* demands.

14. Don't try to teach him too much at one time. If you do, he'll get all mixed up and will resent the next lesson. A chock-full agenda usually produces nothing.

15. Don't be afraid to admit a mistake. But do it in a dignified fashion—don't start crawling. Silly as this sounds, I heard of many such cases. Your pet wants to be able to look up to you and he doesn't want an owner who acts like a dishrag.

16. Don't own a pet unless you're prepared to take care of it. This may appear to be far removed from two-way conversations, but it isn't! Your pet will refuse to cooperate if he feels that you are neglecting him. And remember: animals can be very stubborn.

17. **Don't feel that pet communication is a sometime thing.** Be prepared to stick with it and display optimism until it produces results. If you're lackadaisical about this enterprise, you can expect that your animal will soon respond similarly.

18. **Don't concentrate only on your pet's body movements.** Verbal signals are also very important. Learn to identify them. A good way is by jotting them down in your notebook.

19. **Don't give your pet a ridiculous-sounding name.** He may not resent the actual name, but he will sense that people smirk when they call him and that fact can make him super-sensitive. Why ask for trouble when its's so easy to avoid? The name of a mature pet can be changed, although this requires a great deal of work on your part. You really have to bear down and use a new name often—almost every sentence should contain a mention of it. After a while, you can let up. But until you're certain that he responds to the new name you have to keep working at it—and ask the other members of your family to help out.

20. **Don't expect too much from your pet.** But be prepared for times when his repertoire will fool you. Recently, I chuckled at a tongue-in-cheek story told to me by a Boston veterinarian. It seems that Duke, a three-year-old English setter, possessed a very high IQ,

and the proud owner sent the dog off to college. Home for the spring vacation, Duke admitted he had done badly in history and economics, but added haughtily, "I did do rather well in foreign languages."

"Okay," conceded the owner. "Say something in a foreign language."

The dog said, "*Miaow.*"

CHAPTER XIII

Pet Communication Dictionary

Household pet owners will find the following listings helpful in carrying on effective two-way conversations. Some of these commonly used verbal and non-verbal signals are discussed in earlier sections, but this separate chart is more complete as well as being handier for everyday use. I was fortunate in securing the help of leading veterinarians, trainers, and alert pet owners in preparing this basic primer.

At the moment some of these words or phrases may not be in your pet's repertoire, but all of them can definitely be mastered. All it usually takes is a bit of conditioning and patience. Some words, sounds, or signals may have a different meaning in the case of your pet because animals, like humans, vary widely and their personalities and abilities appear very diverse. That is why careful observation is so necessary and why I appeal to you to get to know your pet intimately—superior animal communication depends on it.

I also suggest that you teach one word—or phrase—at

a time, and never run your sessions for longer than fifteen minutes; psychologists have discovered that animals grow weary of a longer period. A successful performance should always pay off in instant praise and a physical reward for the animal—*something the animal likes, not what you think he should like.* A simple biscuit will often work wonders. After several weeks of practice sessions the words will become a natural part of the pet's accustomed routine, and praise alone is usually sufficient.

Although you may regard some of the expressions listed below as being too obvious and familiar, the professionals whom I consulted urged me to include even the *familiar* terms. Captain Arthur Haggerty, director of one of the largest trainer schools in the country, had a typical comment: "Where pets are concerned," he said, "constant repetition is of tremendous benefit to both the owner and the animal. Also, I've often seen the owner take for granted what he thought the animal was saying—and, too often, the interpretation was totally wrong!"

Herewith the list of frequently used expressions:

Dogs

Dog to owner (non-verbal).

1. **"Don't tease me."** The dog lies down on the floor several feet away from you, but still within sight. His tail is held between the legs and ears are down. He opens and shuts his mouth, making loud clicking sounds

that almost sound as if he's saying, **"Clark Kent, Clark Kent."**

2. **"I feel apprehensive and aggressive at the same time."** Dogs are frequently in this mood of indecision. The head and tail are alternately raised and lowered. When they are up it usually signifies aggression; down means apprehension.

3. **"I'm satisfied with everything."** He pulls his lips back and one corner of his mouth is formed into a small crease that makes him appear to be smiling. His ears are lowered and his eyelids are half closed. He often barks shrilly and thereby confuses the owner. Barking can be an expression of pleasure to convey the message that the dog has learned to deal with a specific difficult situation.

4. **"Comfort me, I'm afraid."** Ears are flattened against his head and again the dog appears to be grinning. However, if you look closely you see that the "grin" is slightly different from the one above—his lips are set wider apart. If the fear increases the grin grows into a deep scowl.

5. **"I forgive you, let's be friends."** He barks excitedly and moves close to you. He usually sits down and tucks his tail tightly between his legs. The tongue is pulled in and out. His eyes are opened wide.

6. **"I'm interested, but I have some doubts."** Dog lowers and raises his ears, head, and tail. When they are

in the down position it usually means he's still doubtful; when they are up he is sure.

7. "This is exciting." His tail is up and he wags it violently. Ears are usually up, but occasionally they move up and down. (Often the owner thinks the wagging tail is merely a friendly gesture and soon finds out otherwise.)

8. "You can do anything to me—within reason." One of the hind legs is raised and you can plainly see the underside. Dog's tail is tucked against his chest; his eyes are narrowed, ears are pulled back and mouth is stretched into what looks like a grin. Suddenly, he starts rolling on the ground.

9. "Come play with me." Tail is up, ears are back, the front of the body is lower than the rear end. He touches his paw to his mouth and often communicates his desire to play by opening his mouth as if he's about to start panting. Sometimes, he actually pants.

10. "I like you very much." The dog's tail is out about three-quarter length and he wags it from side to side. Ears are up and he appears to be grinning. He may nuzzle against you if you're standing or put his head in your lap if you are sitting.

11. "Watch where you're going, you just stepped on me." Eyes appear to be glowing, ears point out. Back end is lower than front. Dog makes a yelping sound— short and shrill. His message is similar to a person saying: "It's all right this time, but from now on you'd better watch out."

12. **"It's okay to have children around, but why do they have to annoy me?"** Dogs are usually gentle with children, but the animals resent unkind treatment from them. Often they escape by running to some inaccessible place, but most times they stay and stoically accept the roughness and inconsideration. The dog usually reflects the pain—ears are flattened against head, lips seem to be wrinkled, and tail is rigid.

13. **"What a nice surprise!"** The dog wags his tail violently. The head is raised and the ears are erect. The lips are pulled down. He emits a loud, vibrating squeal. Also used for greeting a member of family who has been away for a long time.

14. **"Why do you always keep me locked up behind the fence? Sometimes I get the urge to wander."** This is usually triggered by the presence of a strange dog. Your dog's hair appears suddenly to bristle, his ears are down, his tail is tucked between his legs. When the other dog is in sight, your dog snarls and looks at you. He then starts to walk around stiff-legged with his tail and head raised.

15. **"I'm glad you've come home."** He runs toward you, barking excitedly. His tail wags in the high position. As you make contact he becomes more excited and sometimes a few drops of urine appear. If that happens he may suddenly become ashamed and try to divert your attention by rolling over.

16. **"It's time for me to be fed."** He stares fixedly at the refrigerator, closet or wherever the dog's food is kept. Some dogs stare at the feeding bowl if it's within sight. Ears are usually up and body sways slightly. Sometimes a dog rubs his eyes with his forepaw.

17. **"I am in total agreement."** Ears are cocked, the face is tilted to the left, and usually this is accompanied by several short, clipped barks.

18. **"No, I don't agree."** Ears are down, the face is tilted to the right side, and this time the barks are high-pitched.

19. **"I don't feel so well."** The dog suddenly appears listless and doesn't respond to the owner's call. He may lie down in a dark corner and appear to be sleeping, but he isn't—if you look closely you can detect signs of his being awake. His mouth may be open. Sometimes he will actually move his paw to the painful area: paw to mouth indicating a sore throat or paw to stomach to tell you that he has a bellyache.

20. **"I'm in heat."** This message is sent in a great variety of ways. However, some common signals are: the lifting of the tail; suddenly becoming moody; frequent barking. Stains are often visible. Some owners told me that their bitches communicate their being in heat by suddenly shredding newspaper or knocking over sugar bowls. One woman said she always knew the dog was in heat because the dog would start yodeling what sounded like the first line of "Oh, Susannah."

21. **"Please, no bath today—anything but that!"** The dog's eyes are opened wide as he looks at you pleadingly. He refuses to remove them from your face, but seems to be aware of your every move. The dog appears to be very listless and wags his tail languidly. If you fail to give him the answer he desires—usually within seconds—he will try to hide in some inaccessible place.

22. **"What did you buy at the store?"** As soon as you come into the house carrying a package he becomes very affectionate. He will lick your hand and rub up against you. His head is held up high as he stares at a parcel. Often he will prance on both legs and as he does this he may lose his balance and suddenly fall over backwards.

23. **"This is hard to do—I could sure use some help."** He wags his tail violently, ears are up, and eyes are half closed. He will issue sharp, low barks. The dog will suddenly flop to the floor, then a moment later get up and run in zigzag fashion around the room. The barking usually becomes more intense.

24. **"I'd like to go for a ride in the car."** This request is usually very unexpected; quite suddenly he will squat on the floor and almost immediately jump up and start to bark. He rapidly moves his tail and ears. Sometimes the barking turns into howling. If you normally wear gloves or a hat or some other specific garment when driving he will squat in front of the closet, shake his head vigorously, and move his front paws. One woman told me that her poodle whirled his paw in circular

fashion suggesting a steering wheel. The squatting often resembles the old-fashioned courtesy of an inviting bow.

25. **"I want to go out for a walk."** The dog fetches the leash with his mouth, brings it over to the owner, then stands in front of the door and occasionally barks. If that doesn't work he will resort to non-verbal communication and run from door to owner and back to the door. He will repeat this performance many times or until he thinks owner is aware of his request.

26. **"What's that?"** There may be a reflection at the window or you may suddenly move. He shakes his head and grows taut. The hair on his body rises. The face is tilted and he wags his tail. Some owners maintain that as the volume of the tail wagging increases his face is tilted to the right side.

27. **"Oh, what's the use—things look so bad."** This mood is easy to detect because the dog looks so dejected. The ears are flat to the head, the eyes seem to sag. The dog doesn't appear to have any tail—it is concealed by one of the legs. He is usually very silent and solemn—seldom does he resort to vocal language.

28. **"I'd like some of that, it sure looks good."** The dog stares directly at your plate while drooling. He may gaze both at you and the plate in rapid succession. His ears are alternately raised and lowered while he watches. Every minute or so he moves a little closer and soon his nose is touching the table. If you offer him

something other than what you're eating he will probably scorn it and issue angry, staccato barks.

29. **"Don't invite those pesky people over again."** His tail is rigid and it is usually held straight out, but careful observation will reveal that he is wagging it ever so slightly. The ears are at right angles to his head, which is slightly bent. Often he will butt into your legs if you're seated.

30. **"I think you ought to stay in tonight."** The body sways from left to right. The eyes are opened wide and the ears are up. His tail is tucked between his legs. Often he will flop down on the floor and appear to be exhausted. Sometimes, a slight discharge of saliva is noticed.

Owner to dog (non-verbal).

1. **"No!"** Owners use many ways to communicate this negative command. The most popular are: clapping of hands, pounding a table, stamping a foot, or flicking a light switch on and off.

2. **"Do be quiet!"** The forefinger is placed against the lips and the eyes are slightly widened.

3. **"Stop doing that!"** When in another room or out of sight, loudly tap or bang on the nearest object.

4. **"I want you to cease begging!"** This is another

time for sudden noise, and for some unknown reason the noise to discourage begging or taking food off the table works best when it is high-pitched. Banging a spoon on an aluminum frying pan usually makes the right sound.

5. **"Come here this minute!"** Snap fingers or start to whistle. This is often accompanied by moving the fingers toward you. Another frequently used method is to swing your right arm loosely. Then bring it up to your left shoulder.

6. **"Your food is ready."** Spoon is banged against food dish or dish is rattled firmly. Banging on the refrigerator door often serves the same purpose.

7. **"Are you finished?"** Stare at the dog and move your head slowly upward. Even though the dog's back may be facing you he seems to have eyes in back of his head.

8. **"Down!"** Many signs are used for this command, but the most effective one is firmly, but gently, to push down on the dog's back and with the other hand point to the ground.

9. **"I like you."** This is best expressed by gently scratching and petting the dog in areas that you know he enjoys having touched.

10. **"Move a little faster."** Your own speeded-up actions will soon convince him that he should do likewise. Owners have found that a swift mopping of the floor or

a hurried job of putting away the dishes or books gives him the idea of haste.

11. **"Relax, be at ease."** Both hands are extended and your palms are opened; you move them to and fro. Your eyes are often widened and lips puckered.

12. **"I'm not angry with you."** You may not have time to convince the dog by petting him, but a quick look, a lowering of the eyes, and a brief smile will often be sufficient.

13. **"I am displeased."** Instead of lowering the eyes, continue to stare and shake your head vigorously. The eyes are widened and lips tightened.

14. **"Don't bother me now."** Move about four feet away from the dog and point your finger. Move it rapidly, keeping it stiff and in a horizontal position. If the dog comes toward you, shoo him away and repeat this performance. After a few times he should get the message.

15. **"The house isn't a toilet!"** You have often been told not to scold the dog unless you catch him in the act, because he won't connect his performance with your disapproval if his misbehavior happened some time earlier. There is some disagreement on this point, but all trainers agree that making some sudden noise if you do find him urinating or defecating will be beneficial. (You might want to accompany this with a vocal "NO!" But be sure to sound as if you mean it.) Then take the dog outside to finish. When he does, praise him.

16. **"Chase the ball and bring it to me."** Toss the ball, then flick your wrist in a semi-circle and point your index finger toward your chest.

17. **"Guess what I have for you?"** He loves to play games, especially ones that you invent. Simply hiding an object and having him locate it will cause him great delight.

18. **"That is not the proper way to do it."** You take him out on the leash and he suddenly does something that you think he shouldn't (be reasonable). You want to communicate your displeasure. Now is the time for the corrective jerk. Jerk the leash firmly to the right. Once is sufficient—don't overdo it!

19. **"Stop removing the garbage from the can."** If you catch him in the act, look stern and violently shake your head from side to side. Banish him to another room or outside. All of these actions should show him your displeasure. But if they don't work it's time to get out your training leash quickly and use the corrective jerk again. Show him the scattered garbage and jerk.

20. **"I need some cheering up."** This is one time you don't have to use any specific sign as your natural expression will usually be sufficient for him to interpret. Dogs constantly observe facial expressions and body movements. They are extremely sensitive to all human moods and will often reflect them.

A fourteen-year-old youth recently told me, "My father had just died and my mother was grieving terribly. Fan-Fan, our French poodle, sensed how Mother felt and promptly offered his condolences. His face had a very sad expression as he jumped into her lap and 'petted' her instead of it always being the other way around. It helped tremendously."

Owner to dog (verbal).

Dr. John Paul Scott, professor of psychology at Bowling Green University, says, "A trained dog can learn to discriminate between as many as seventy-five and one hundred individual words."

Here are the most common ones I discovered:

1. baby
2. bath
3. bad
4. ball
5. bark
6. bed
7. bird
8. biscuit
9. bone
10. book
11. bowl (pertaining to food; however, some dogs are familiar with word when applied to game)
12. boy
13. can (applies to food)
14. car (for some reason the Volkswagen is recognized best)
15. cat
16. chair
17. child

18. cold
19. come
20. cookie
21. cracker
22. crawl
23. crib
24. daddy
25. dinner
26. dog
27. door
28. doorbell
29. drop
30. eat
31. feed
32. fetch
33. food
34. friend
35. garbage
36. garden
37. get
38. girl
39. go
40. good
41. head
42. heel
43. hell
44. hide
45. horn
46. hot
47. house
48. hurry
49. I, me (owner)
50. jeep

51. lady
52. leash
53. leave
54. lick
55. magazine
56. mailman
57. man
58. mommy
59. mood
60. name (his own and others)
61. newspaper
62. no
63. off
64. out
65. piano
66. puppy
67. quiet
68. rain
69. ring (sound)
70. run
71. shake
72. shoe
73. shoot
74. sick
75. sing
76. sit
77. sleep
78. sofa
79. stay
80. stick
81. store
82. street
83. snow

84. swim
85. tail
86. telephone
87. tree
88. umbrella
89. up
90. vet
91. walk
92. wander
93. water
94. weather
96. wet
97. whisper
98. whiskey (martini, cocktail, etc.)
99. work
100. yes

Dog to owner (verbal).

Dogs communicate mainly in silence and their vocal
"words" only have significance when you are aware of
their accompanying body language. However, the following six sounds are used by many dogs:

1. **"There's an intruder at the door."** Deep, continuous growls to warn the owner of an unexpected
"guest."

2. **"Wow, that sure hurts!"** The dog suddenly experiences pain and emits short and shrill sounds that are
referred to as "yelping."

3. **"Stay away, this is my territory!"** Another dog suddenly invades what your dog considers his private domain. He shows his displeasure by repeated snarling.

4. **"Play it again, Sam."** The dog draws his lower lip down while he hears the playing of music. Suddenly, he joins in by beginning to howl. (If a dog howls persistently a vet should be consulted.)

5. **"My master's gone away."** If the owner is gone for the day or longer, the lonely dog starts to whine.

6. **"The prodigal son returns."** When a favorite member of the family returns, the dog may show his delight and surprise by suddenly squealing.

Cats

Although cats express themselves with great feeling and resourcefulness through body language, many of the animal behaviorists I consulted said that a feline's repertoire is slightly smaller than a dog's.

Cat to owner (non-verbal).

1. **"Welcome home."** The tail stands straight up. The head is lowered and almost touches the ground. Solicits stroking and petting from the recent arrival. Occasionally, the cat rolls on the ground.

2. **"I want to be fed."** Jumps up on the kitchen

counter or stands in front of the food closet or refriger-ator and miaows. The tail is up, but bent. The ears are up. Often the cat crouches and leans forward. If there is no immediate response the cat will pace back and forth. If there is still no action he will claw at the door con-taining the food. Occasionally, he will rub against the owner's leg as he miaows.

3. **"Something seems to be threatening me."** The cat swipes at nearest thing to him—rarely a person. He growls deeply and often rubs his head against a chair or sofa.

4. **"What do you want?"** Runs to you with ears pointed upward and the tail standing straight up. He appears to be concentrating on the sound you are making. Cats possess a mobile external ear (called *pinna)*—it is used to collect sound waves.

5. **"I'm curious about that thingamajig."** Closes eyes, but opens mouth and sniffs. This seems to be a very common occurrence.

6. **"I want to go outside."** He runs just a few inches ahead of you. Frequently he is so close that you have to avoid stepping on him. His legs are moving so rapidly that at times he looks like he's kicking a football. If you suddenly halt he stares directly into your eyes. His jaw appears to be fully opened.

7. **"I guess it's all right, don't fret."** If you accident-ally step on him, he will rub against your leg to show

you that no hard feelings exist. His eyes are opened wide and his whiskers appear to be shaking.

8. "Everything's at peace with me and the world." He suddenly goes all cuddly. His tail is curled around his body. The ears are back and the eyes keep opening and closing. Sometimes he shows his contentment by making his tail stand straight up.

9. "There's a mouse hiding in that little hole." He lies down in front of the hole and stares fixedly at it. All four paws are tucked under his body, ears are slightly bent and tail curls outward. Every thirty seconds or so one of cat's front paws is thrust into hole. Hunger has nothing to do with the desire for mouse-catching. As a matter of fact, a well-fed cat is likely to catch more mice than a hungry one.

10. "You call that food?" He shakes his paw at the food in his dish. He does this vigorously, using an up-and-down motion. Then he backs away from the un-eaten food. A few seconds later he returns, but still refuses to eat. Often he will miaow while doing this.

11. "Let's play!" He starts by running around the room and then singles you out. If you are sitting he may jump into your lap, stay there for a moment, and then hop onto a table. Moments later he will jump down and start the procedure over again. His tail is curled into a U position. He may get on his side and roll over several times.

12. **"I've had enough play and want to stop."** He stretches lazily and then moves to some inaccessible place, perhaps under the bed, or climbs on top of a very high bookcase. He will claw playfully, but firmly, if you attempt to get him. One of the most fascinating things about a cat is his sense of timing—he knows when enough is enough.

13. **"I can tell that you're depressed and need some cheering up."** He will crouch in front of you and stare directly into your eyes. His ears move quickly up and down. He may miaow gently, but often he remains mute. He hopes that you will pick him up. Once in your lap he will appear to be sleeping, but suddenly his tongue will lick your hand and face.

14. **"That's a good show you're watching on television."** Jumps on top of the set and promptly jumps off. He may do this several times, but he's not doing it to annoy you; he just hasn't made up his mind if he really wants to view the show. When he does, he crouches in front of the screen or occasionally will lie backward on top of the set and twist his head downward while he views the show in an inverted position. Cats seem to prefer action shows—they like watching cowboy chases and wrestling matches.

15. **"You've slept enough, it's time to rise and shine!"** He may pull the covers off you—there's nothing subtle about his performance. Or he might stand at the foot of the bed and simply stare. Owners say that they can't be oblivious to this staring—it soon makes them pop out of bed and start preparing the cat's breakfast.

16. **"The room is cold, turn the heat up."** The tail moves up and down vigorously as he sways his body from side to side. Cats seem to prefer a hot house and will usually miaow loudly until the owner responds with more heat.

17. **"It's raining so hard that you wouldn't even make a dog go out."** He stands staring out of the front door and suddenly his body grows stiff. His ears go up and his mouth is opened wide. Unless you push or carry him out, he won't budge.

18. **"Someone's at the door."** The cat races to the owner and miaows furiously. He looks up and frowns. His pupils grow larger and his ears wiggle back and forth.

19. **"I'm jealous."** He lets out a loud howl and quickly scurries off. Returns in a few seconds (he may be jealous of another cat's presence) to see if his competition is still there. If so he will hurriedly leave again.

20. **"I'm coming in season."** If the female cat has not been spayed she will seek affection from her owner, come to be stroked. At this time she will often rub against the owner with much purring and sad eyes.

21. **"Do you mind repeating that?"** The cat is in upright position with his tail curled behind him. Eyes are riveted to your face and his head rotates slightly, but he continues to stare. Occasionally, the mouth is opened wide and you can plainly see his teeth.

22. **"I admit I'm jealous."** If a cat was facing away from you he will turn in your direction and crouch on the floor. His head is slightly cocked, ears are halfway up, and eyes blink rapidly as he sits and sulks. Longtime owners told me that they can always tell when a cat gets jealous by noticing the distinct signs of nervous strain on his face.

23. **"Don't bother me. I'm thinking."** His paws are tucked in and tail is curled around body. Head is up and tips of ears appear to be bent. Eyes open and close. When they are open the cat appears to be staring at the ceiling.

24. **"I feel so stupid."** The cat raises his front paws as he begins kneading. After a moment or two the kneading becomes more rapid. He drools and swipes at imaginary bugs on the wall. His head bobs up and down.

25. **"You think I'm only a cat, but I've got feelings, too!"** The pupils in his eyes suddenly dilate. He appears to be frowning and often will shake his head at you. If you call him he will refuse to come. If you attempt to pick him up he will grow limp and scoot out of your hands. The best thing to do is to offer praise and start petting.

Owner to cat (non-verbal).

The experts whom I consulted told me that most of the expressions that appear in the "owner to dog, non-verbal" section apply equally to cats. Read them carefully and try them—you'll soon agree. However, you are cautioned that in order to be successful, a large amount of patience is required. One cat owner told me, "My cat was the most obstinate creature I ever encountered. She pretended not to understand anything I told her and I almost gave up all hope of ever reaching her. However, I kept trying and one day, like a miracle, she started listening to me. It sure was worth the wait!"

Owner to cat (verbal).

Ms. Gillette Grilhé, a graduate of the Sorbonne and a recognized authority on cats, has written extensively about man's relationship with the cat. She says, "The cat's vocabulary contains sixty-three sounds." Other researchers told me that the figure is much higher. Dr. Milton Kreutzer, an Illinois psychologist, said, "It's well over a hundred. Not only can the cat talk to man, but the cat knows most of the things man says."
Here I offer you a minimum list of my own.

1. away
2. bad
3. ball
4. basement
5. basket
6. beautiful
7. bed
8. bird
9. cage
10. chew

11. chicken
12. clawing
13. climb
14. coat
15. cold
16. comb
17. come
18. counter
19. cover
20. dinner
21. doctor
22. don't
23. dog
24. eat
25. fight
26. fire
27. floor
28. food
29. garbage
30. good
31. grass
32. hat
33. head
34. hungry
35. I, me (owner)
36. kiss
37. kitten
38. lick
39. love
40. milk
41. mouse
42. name (own or others)
43. naughty

44. nice
45. no
46. noise
47. off
48. out
49. phone
50. pill
51. pillow
52. plate
53. play
54. pretty
55. pussy
56. rug
57. sick
58. sleep
59. soap
60. sock, stocking
61. string
62. suitcase
63. sweep
64. television
65. toy
66. turn
67. typewriter
68. under
69. undress
70. vacuum cleaner
71. water
72. where
73. whirl
74. work
75. yes

Cat to owner (verbal).

Although most cats emit more than fifteen distinct sounds they fall into three categories:

1. Miaowing. This is of course the chief sound of the cat and varies in intensity and pitch with every feline. Therefore, it is suggested that the owner carefully study his individual animal to determine what the particular miaow means, since the cat uses it on many, many occasions:

> **"I'm hungry, feed me."**
> **"How about playing with me?"**
> **"I don't feel so well."**
> **"Stop making all that noise!"**
> **"Glad to see you."**

2. Purring. This sound, as everyone knows, is used when the cat is in a state of contentment and joy. However, there are a few times when the feline will purr when in extreme pain, but that is quite rare. No one knows exactly how cats purr, but the sound is unmistakable—it's a low, continuous sound chiefly used when he is in a friendly, relaxed state. Some of its obvious meanings are:

> **"Oh, that scratching felt ever so good."**
> **"I feel so very, very happy."**
> **"You are right—I am indeed a lovely-looking animal."**
> **"That was a delicious meal."**
> **"Thank you for that yummy goodie."**

3. **Hissing.** Whenever a cat is threatened by a dog, or another cat, he will start hissing. If attacked, the hissing becomes louder and louder. When aroused or afraid, the cat will make this sound and behaviorists point out that this happens quite often because the cat is more aggressive than the dog. Even in mating, the male and female will hiss at each other. A hiss may mean:

"**Beware, you have to contend with me!**"
"**This is my territory—keep out!**"
"**You may be bigger, but I'll take you on!**"
"**I'm King of the Mountain and I want everybody to be aware!**"
"**I'll show that cat who's boss!**"

Cat sounds have been classified under three main groups: *Murmur* patterns in a friendly relaxed state; *vowel* patterns that are used when the cat is seeking care or is frustrated when he tries to accomplish something; and *strained intensity* sounds that the cat makes when he attacks, defends or mates.

Examples of the three are:

1. "**I like being petted.**" The cat makes a purring sound during this occurrence.

2. "**Feed me.**" He emits a more articulated sound when demanding food. The sound is often referred to as "miaowing."

3. "**I'll show that cat who's boss!**" Your cat starts

hissing and screaming when he is annoyed or threatened.

Birds

Birds come in such a great variety that it is very difficult to generalize. Nevertheless, the following three signals are almost universal:

1. **"I suddenly feel alarmed."** The bird may issue a sharp, insistent cry. This call is very different from his usual repertoire and as he becomes more alarmed the cry becomes sharper and increases in volume. He flies wildly around his cage and, when you stand next to it, his frenzy becomes more apparent.

2. **"I'm lonely and want company."** His head is tilted to one side and his neck seems to be outstretched. He sings a tune that is very simple, almost consisting of two notes. As you approach, he often leaves his perch and flies in your direction.

3. **"I'm over here, remember me."** His neck is puffed out and he struts back and forth. This time his song might be compared to a human's whistle that contains a slight trill.

Horses

Horse to owner (verbal).

1. "Hey, isn't it time for dinner?"

The horse will emit a loud whinny that sounds like, "*Henh, henh, henh.*" Learning to recognize this communication is a good way to start understanding horses because it is so obvious.

2. "Oh, here you are! Glad to see you!"

A soft nicker, sounding like, "*Humph, humph, humph,*" is often given when the owner approaches. There still is controversy over the ability of a horse to recognize any human by sight. Many scientists now believe that any recognition is more likely to be the result of the horse's sense of smell, which is much more acute than his eyesight.

Horse to owner (non-verbal).

1. "I'm waiting to be told what to do."

Ears flicking back and forth tell the rider that the horse is willing to cooperate and feels very good. (Willi Schultheis, the outstanding German dressage rider and trainer, said, "You must never underrate the importance of the horse's ears—they are excellent barometers for determining the horse's mood or attitude.")

2. "That looks (or sounds) interesting."

You are out for a ride and notice that one of the

horse's ears is turned back and the other one leans forward. This usually means that he sees something curious up ahead—a squirrel or a pheasant—but nothing that presents any peril.

3. "Look out, there's danger coming up!"

If a horse's ears suddenly shoot forward, then you'd better watch out for some unexpected hazard—a very-low-hanging branch, falling rocks, a sharp swerve in the trail. . . .

4. "It may not be spring, but suddenly I've got spring fever."

When his ears are upright but relaxed, it's a sure sign that he's not concentrating. An American Horse Show executive told me, "First the ears and then the entire body seem to become limp—rag-dolly."

5. "I'm about to do something that you won't like."

The horse's ears come down flat against his head. When they do, it's generally a signal that he's about to create havoc. He may suddenly buck. So be prepared!

6. "Why don't you learn how to ride?"

This admonition is communicated in many ways, but one of the most frequent signals is this: the horse takes several mincing steps, fights the bit and refuses to move. He may be telling you that you're riding him too severely and with too heavy a hand.

7. "There's only one boss and I'm it!"

Although many people claim that a horse isn't intelligent, here is evidence to the contrary: when the rider is a young child, the animal will take advantage of that fact and often stop to eat grass. Behaviorists say that the horse deliberately wants to show that he is the stronger of the two.

8. "Don't fret, I'm just being playful."

When you want a horse to trot or canter, he starts jigging instead. He also reveals his gaiety by keeping his tail up, tossing his head around and bucking. No need for concern—unless the bucking hurts your butt.

9. "Here comes a kick!"

The horse's tail is tucked between the legs. In the case of other animals this may signify slinking cowardice, but with a horse it's usually a sign that a kick is imminent. Watch out!

10. "I feel exhausted."

Sweating is a very good indication of a horse's fitness, and should always be considered as a communication. It is quite natural for a horse in superior physical shape to sweat profusely after a brisk workout, but he soon gets over it. A horse in really soft condition will sweat more readily and take much longer to return to normal. Sweating should guide the owner in determining the amount of work or play that the animal can stand.

11. "I'm a nervous wreck!"

The horse will wave his head back and forth, and sway from side to side. He may also pace around his stall and never seem to locate a comfortable spot.

12. "Old age seems to be creeping up on me."

His withers become more prominent, the lower lip hangs down and his teeth appear to be getting longer —horses' teeth grow throughout their lives. (The theory about determining a horse's age by looking at his teeth is valid, but at times only partly accurate, since much depends on what food the animal has been given as a steady diet. A year of a horse's life is equivalent to three of a human's.)

13. "I'm getting angrier by the minute!"
The horse will swish his tail, roll his eyes and push his ears flat back. Often he lowers his head and appears to be extremely rigid. This behavior is a sure sign of discomfort or loss of temper. Benny "Blintzes" Schaefer, an inveterate racetrack visitor, told me with assurance: "When I see a horse do those things I know for sure that he won't come in the money, so I lay off him. Another dead giveaway is when the nag starts pawing the ground with his right leg and makes a loud grunt—kind of like, 'Ughchoop!' A horse tells you lots of things, but you got to look real sharp to get what he's saying!"

John Tyler, the tenth President of the United States, did just that—and he found the results very worthwhile. White House employees revealed that the President constantly carried on conversations with General, his favorite steed. When the horse died, President Tyler had a monument placed on his grave in Sherwood Forest, Virginia. It reads: "Here lies the body of my good horse, the General. For years he bore me around the circuit of my law practice and all the time he never made a mistake. Would that his master could say the same—John Tyler."

Bibliography

Books

Adams, Richard. *Watership Down*. New York: Macmillan, 1974.

Armstrong, Edward A. *A Study of Bird Song*. New York: Dover Publications, 1973.

Borgese, Elisabeth Mann. *The Language Barrier—Beasts and Men*. New York: Holt, Rinehart and Winston, 1968.

Brooke, Geoffrey. *Horse Lovers*. New York: Charles Scribner, 1937.

Campbell, Judith. *Horses and Ponies*. New York: Grosset & Dunlap, 1971.

Clement, Herb. *Zoo Man*. New York: Macmillan, 1969.

Cohen, Daniel. *Talking with the Animal*. New York: Dodd, Mead & Company, 1971.

Cosgrove, Margaret. *Messages and Voices*. New York: Dodd, Mead & Company, 1974.

Darwin, Charles. *The Variation of Plants and Animals Under Domestication*. London: International Publications Service, 1868.

Disston, Harry. *Know About Horses*. New York: Devin-Adair, 1961.

Eustace, M., and Towe, T. *The Royal Cat of Siam*. London: Pelham, 1968.

Evans, William. *Communication in the Animal World*. New York: Thomas Y. Crowell Company, 1968.

Bibliography

Fast, Julius. *Body Language.* New York: M. Evans & Co., Inc., 1970.

Fichtelius, K. E., and Sjolander, S. *Smarter Than Man?* New York: Random House, 1972.

Fox, Michael W. *Understanding Your Dog.* New York: Coward, McCann and Geoghegan, 1971.

———. *Understanding Your Cat.* New York: Coward, McCann and Geoghegan, 1974.

———. *Canine Behavior.* Springfield, Ill.: Charles C. Thomas, 1965.

———. *Behavior of Wolves, Dogs and Related Canines.* New York: Harper & Row, 1971.

Gautier, Jean. *A Priest and His Dog.* New York: Macmillan Company, 1957.

Gilbert, Bil. *How Animals Communicate.* New York: Pantheon Books, 1966.

Grilhé, Gillette. *The Cat and Man.* New York: G. P. Putman's Sons, 1974.

Hays, S. C. *The Ape in Our House.* New York: Harper and Bros., 1951.

Hope, Charles E. G. *The Horseman's Manual.* New York: Charles Scribner's Sons, 1974.

Johnson, Pat. *Meet the Horse.* New York: Grosset & Dunlap, 1967.

Koenig, Lilli. *Studies in Animal Behavior.* New York: Thomas Y. Crowell, 1967.

Lewinsohn, Richard. *Animals, Man and Myth.* New York: Harper and Bros., 1954.

Levinson, Boris. *Pets and Human Development.* Springfield, Ill.: Charles C. Thomas, 1972.

Lilly, John C. *The Mind of the Dolphin.* New York: Doubleday and Company, Inc., 1967.

Lockley, Ronald. *The Private Life of the Rabbit.* New York: Macmillan, 1973.

Bibliography

Lorenz, Konrad. *King Solomon's Ring.* New York: Thomas Y. Crowell Company, 1952.

———. *Man Meets Dog.* London: Penguin Books, 1964.

Metcalf, C. *Cats.* London: Paul Hamlyn, 1967.

Milne, Louis and Margery. *The Balance of Nature.* New York: Alfred A. Knopf, Inc., 1960.

———. *The Senses of Animals and Men.* New York: Atheneum, 1972.

Manning, O: *Extraordinary Cats.* London: Michael Joseph, 1967.

Putnam, Peter. *Triumph of the Seeing Eye.* New York: Harper & Row, 1963.

Rice, B. *The Other End of the Leash: The American Way with Pets.* London: Angus and Robertson, 1968.

Robbins, Jhan, and Fisher, David. *How to Make and Break Habits: Behavior Modification.* New York: Peter H. Wyden, 1973.

Scott, John Paul. *Animal Behavior.* Chicago: University of Chicago Press, 1958.

———, and Fuller, J. S. *Genetics and Social Behavior of the Dog.* Chicago: University of Chicago Press, 1965.

Self, Margaret Cabell. *The Horseman's Encyclopedia.* New York: Arco, 1963.

Siegal, Mordecai, and Margolis, Matthew. *Good Dog, Bad Dog.* New York: Holt, Rinehart and Winston, 1973.

———. *Underdog.* New York: Stein & Day, 1974.

Sparks, John. *Bird Behavior.* New York: Grosset & Dunlap, Inc., 1970.

Steinuit, Robert. *The Dolphin, Cousin to Man.* New York: Sterling Publishing Company, 1968.

Bibliography

Stefferud, Alfred, ed. *Birds in Our Lives.* New York: Arco, 1971.

Stoneridge, M. A. *A Horse of Your Own.* New York: Doubleday & Company, 1968.

Thompson, Ernest Seton. *Wild Animals I Have Known.* New York: Charles Scribner's Sons, 1901.

Tomkins, Peter, and Bird, Christopher. *The Secret Life of Plants.* New York: Harper & Row, 1973.

Trench, Charles Chenuix. *History of Horsemanship.* London: Longman, 1970.

von Frisch, Karl. *Bees: Their Vision, Chemical Senses and Languages.* Ithaca, New York: Cornell University Press, 1960.

———. *The Dancing Bees.* New York: Harcourt, Brace and Company, 1955.

Whitney, Leon. *The Complete Book of Pet Care.* New York: Doubleday & Company, 1950.

Williams, Moyra. *Horse Psychology.* New York: Arco, 1969.

Periodicals

Duncan, S., Jr. "Nonverbal Communication." *Psychiatric Bulletin,* No. 72, pp. 118–157.

Fleming, Joyce Dudney. "The State of the Apes." *Psychology Today,* January 1974, pp. 31–50.

Fouts, R. S. "Acquisition and Testing of Gestural Signs." *Science,* June 1, 1973, pp. 978–980.

Fox, Michael. "Everything You Always Wanted to Know About Your Dog." *Washington University Magazine,* Winter 1972.

Gardner, R. A. and B. T. "Teaching Sign Language to a Chimpanzee." *Science,* 1969, pp. 664–672.

Bibliography

Griffin, D. R. "Sensory Physiology and the Orientation of Animals." *American Scientist,* 1953, pp. 209–244.

Herrnstein, Richard J. "In Defense of Bird Brains." *Atlantic Monthly,* September 1965.

Klopfer, F. Dudley. "Scientific View of Rarey." *American Heritage,* April 1969.

Lorenz, Konrad, F. de Towarnicki. "Talk With Konrad Lorenz. *New York Times Magazine,* July 5, 1970.

Marler, P. "Animal Communication Signals." *Science,* 1967, pp. 769–774.

McCarthy, T. "A Man Who Could Talk to Horses." *American Heritage,* April 1969.

Premack, David. "The Education of Sarah." *Psychology Today,* September 1970, pp. 54–58.

Rumbaugh, D. M. "Reading and Sentence Completion by a Chimpanzee." *Science,* November 15, 1973.

Trotter, R. J. "I Talk to the Animals." *Science News,* June 2, 1973, pp. 360–361.

Whitney, L. F. *McCall's,* October 1969, pp. 70ff.

Wilson, E. O. "Animal Communication." *Scientific American,* September 1972.

The Chronicle of the Horse, numerous back issues.

Phonograph Records

The Language and Music of the Wolves. Narrated by Robert Redford for *National History Magazine.* Tonsil Records.

Virginia Belmont's Famous Singing and Talking Birds. Virginia Belmont Enterprises.

DATE DUE

OCT 0 3 2006		